VAGINA
PROBLEMS

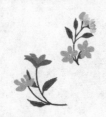

VAGINA PROBLEMS

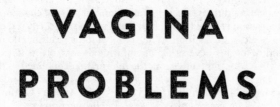

*Endometriosis,
Painful Sex,
and Other
Taboo Topics*

Lara Parker

ST. MARTIN'S GRIFFIN
NEW YORK

The information in this book is not intended to replace the advice of the reader's own physician or other medical professional. You should consult a medical professional in matters relating to health, especially if you have existing medical conditions, and before starting, stopping, or changing the dose of any medication you are taking. Individual readers are solely responsible for their own health care decisions. The author and the publisher do not accept responsibility for any adverse effects individuals may claim to experience, whether directly or indirectly, from the information contained in this book.

First published in the United States by St. Martin's Griffin, an imprint of St. Martin's Publishing Group

www.stmartins.com

Interior photograph: floral pattern © Loric/Shutterstock.com

Designed by Devan Norman

Library of Congress Cataloging-in-Publication Data

Names: Parker, Lara (Writer and editor), author.
Title: Vagina problems : endometriosis, painful sex, and other taboo topics / Lara Parker.
Description: First edition. | New York : St. Martin's Griffin, [2020]
Identifiers: LCCN 2020024208 | ISBN 9781250240682 (trade paperback) | ISBN 9781250240699 (ebook)
Subjects: LCSH: Parker, Lara (Writer and editor)—Health. | Endometriosis—Patients. | Endometriosis—Diagnosis. | Women—Health and hygiene.
Classification: LCC RG483.E53 P37 2020 | DDC 618.1—dc23
LC record available at https://lccn.loc.gov/2020024208

Our books may be purchased in bulk for promotional, educational, or business use. Please contact your local bookseller or the Macmillan Corporate and Premium Sales Department at 1-800-221-7945, extension 5442, or by email at MacmillanSpecialMarkets@macmillan.com.

First Edition: 2020

10 9 8 7 6 5 4 3 2 1

For anyone who has ever felt at war against their own body

Contents

VAGINA
PROBLEMS

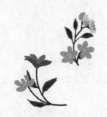

Introduction:
Welcome to the World of Vagina Problems

Vaginas. More than 50 percent of the population has one, but for some reason we're not talking about them much. Sure, they're sometimes mentioned in a magazine or on TV, but we're not talking about them the way we should be. We're not talking about the fact that an estimated 176 million people worldwide live with endometriosis, and around one in ten people with vaginas will experience some sort of vaginal or pelvic pain in their lifetime. We're not talking about painful sex, or painful orgasms, or periods that are so debilitating they keep you home from work or school. That's what we should be talking about.

I have Vagina Problems. I say Vagina Problems because if I start going into every single thing I've ever been diagnosed with, you'd probably try to close out the screen, even though this is a book. What I'm saying is, this shit gets boring. It's a long list of words that mean nothing to the average person, and it's all a complicated way of saying that my vagina hurts, among other things. For the longest time when filling out paperwork with a new doctor or trying to explain my pain to friends, I would try to keep it really simple. I'd say, "Oh, I have stomach problems." It was always easier than trying to explain what the hell endometriosis or vaginismus is. But as the years passed and the diagnoses kept piling on, I was no longer sure what to say or how to say it. It's not *just* my vagina that hurts. It's my legs, my back, my stomach, my vagina, my bladder. And it's not just endometriosis anymore—it's endometriosis, vaginismus, vulvodynia, vulvar vestibulitis syndrome, overall pelvic floor dysfunction, interstitial cystitis, PMDD, fibrocystic breasts, and probable adenomyosis. And those are just the ones that I've actually been able to get a diagnosis or term for. What the hell are all those words I just wrote? I don't even know half the time, if I'm being honest. And, you know, who wants to hear you list all that stuff in everyday conversation? No one. I promise you. No one.

* * *

Years ago, when I was first diagnosed with endometriosis, I had barely even heard of the damn disease. And I wasn't alone. When I would tell people of my new diagnosis as an explanation for my pain over the past several years, they would meet my eyes with a blank stare. And then they would ask me if I was feeling better yet. No, Carol, I'm not feeling better yet. Do you wanna know why, Carol? Because endometriosis, despite affecting almost two hundred million people worldwide, has no cure. And you know what else, CAROL? Most doctors don't even diagnose it properly or have any idea how to begin to treat the symptoms. Oh, and one more thing, Carol—a chronic illness means that it is, in fact, chronic. I don't have the flu!!!! It's not just gonna go away in the week since you last saw me, Carol!

So for years, in order to avoid the urge to punch five to ten people a week, I continued to just say I had stomach problems and leave it at that. But as the years passed and my pain worsened, I had to figure out new terminology. The pain I was experiencing was certainly not the same as that experienced by someone who ate too much Popeye's chicken and felt bloated. This pain needed to be explained in a way that made people understand why I often had to cancel plans or miss work two to three times a month.

So I began to describe my issues as Vagina Problems. My Vagina Problems meant that my abdomen was swollen 93.7 percent of the time. They meant that sitting down for an extended period would make my vagina burn as if someone had put hot acid on it. They meant that wearing thong underwear was a death sentence, and that drinking anything carbonated felt the same as drinking poison. And these problems also meant that I was in a state of almost constant cramping. And no, I don't mean the types of cramps where you can pop an ibuprofen or two and continue on with your day. We're talking the worst period cramps you've ever experienced, but on an almost daily basis. Oh, and just in case you weren't uncomfortable enough already, Carol—these problems also meant I wasn't able to stand penetration of any kind, and when I *was* able to orgasm, it came with a shooting pain to boot. DO YOU GET IT NOW, CAROL????

When I finally started to open up more about my Vagina Problems, I quickly forgot to be ashamed. I had been living with a sore vagina and abdomen for so long at that point that I forgot that my UPS person or my seventh-grade English teacher might not be accustomed to hearing or reading someone talk about their vagina at all, let alone a vagina that hurt. But it all just came pouring out. I had been quiet about my issues for so long that I no longer had the ability to keep my experiences inside. I started talking. And I told everyone. It got to the point where I was saying "My vagina hurts today" the same way someone might say "I have a headache." And it didn't stop there. I didn't just tell my acquaintances and friends. I tweeted about it. I talked about it on Instagram. I said it out loud in dressing rooms and in grocery stores. I wouldn't shut the fuck up about my vagina then, and I don't plan to now.

When I first started experiencing my Vagina Problems, I was just fourteen years old. My period had recently started, and so did the pain. It hurt everywhere, but especially in my abdomen and vagina. It was constant, but worse around my period. But if I'd learned anything about periods before I even started my own, it was that you didn't talk about that shit. Especially not in front of men. When my period came in with a vengeance right off the bat, I mostly just tried to ignore it. I couldn't understand why my period was making me throw up, pass out, and miss school, or why it wrecked an entire week of my life every month while my friends barely even talked about cramps. I convinced myself that everyone must be feeling what I was feeling and that maybe they were just better at hiding it. I knew that my abdomen hurt pretty much constantly, but I had no idea how to talk about it with anyone. And when I *did* find courage to bring it up to my doctor, she brushed it off and made me feel stupid. "Periods are supposed to hurt," she said. I just began to assume that the pain I was feeling in my body was normal, because I had never heard otherwise.

Then, a couple of years later, when I decided to have sex for the first time, it hurt like hell. I mean, it hurt so bad that it felt like someone was shoving a knife dipped in acid inside my vagina—and I assumed that was normal, too. In high school when my friends would talk about sex, they always said it was going to hurt. It's like some unspoken universal rule: If a woman brings up her first time having sex, you *must* tell her about how it's going to hurt. A couple of years after that, when I got up the courage to try again, I assumed the mind-boggling pain I still felt was normal, too. Despite trying to convince myself that everything I was feeling was no big deal, there was a small voice in the back of my head telling me that maybe it wasn't all okay and maybe something was going on in my body. So back to the doctor I went, only this time to be 1) shamed for being sexually active and 2) told that the pain was totally normal the first couple of times and to use lube, duh!

Little did I know that this was only the beginning of a seven-year journey to find out what was going on in my body. It took multiple doctors, thousands of dollars, and a refusal to take no for an answer to finally gain some sort of understanding of what was causing me so much pain. But not everyone has the money for surgeries or access to different doctors for multiple opinions. On average, it takes seven to ten doctors' visits for someone to be diagnosed with endometriosis. And if they are finally diagnosed they are then given just a small handful of options, most of which cost thousands of dollars or come with hefty side effects, and none of which is a cure. The time to start talking openly and honestly about Vagina Problems is long past due.

So here I am, on the other side, well aware of my Vagina Problems and no longer afraid to talk about them. It's been more than ten years since my Vagina Problems first became a constant in my life, and despite numerous attempts at ridding my body of these illnesses I still have the same pain. I still have doctors not believe me when I tell them my symptoms. People still feel uncomfortable when I bring up my vagina. Viagra is still being easily covered by insurance while people sometimes have to lie and say the physical therapy they are getting for their vagina is actually for their back so that insurance will cover it, and we still don't have anything close to an accessible treatment plan for any of it. Millions of people live with conditions similar to mine, but stigma, shame, and lack of awareness keep us all from talking about and normalizing it.

One of the main reasons that I wanted to write this book was because it is something I wished I had when I was first learning about my own Vagina Problems. Most of the literature I found on the subject was either from medical professionals or written based on medical studies and therefore included a lot of medical jargon that was mostly over my head. There is a place for that type of literature, and books like that can be helpful at times, but that wasn't what I needed. What I needed was a book that told me that I wasn't alone—and one that gave me permission to just be upset about going through this. I didn't want to be told, "Just do this and you will feel better." I wanted to be told, "Hey, you're not alone, it sucks, I'm sorry. Let's know it sucks together."

When you have Vagina Problems, it's hard to think about anything else. And quite honestly, I don't think we should have to. This book is for everyone who has ever experienced *any* kind of Vagina Problems. I hear you. I see you. And I believe you.

1

Is Everyone Having Sex but Me?

I had just (barely) graduated from college in the early summer of 2013 when I received the diagnosis, at the Mayo Clinic, that would change my life in so many ways. Looking back on it all now, years later, it seems sort of odd to remember my diagnoses of vulvodynia and vaginismus—two conditions that contribute to painful sex and overall pain of the vulva and vaginal muscles—as the cherry on top of the cake that finally spun me into a dark oblivion, but that's exactly how it happened. I didn't have a grasp on the depth of endometriosis and the ways in which it could cause chronic pain, and even after I received the diagnosis, it felt like something that was in my past and very much not a part of my present and future. However, I was still in some sort of pain nearly every day.

When I arrived at the Mayo Clinic in Rochester, Minnesota— a twelve-hour drive from where I had grown up in Indiana—I was concerned about my pain. It had been increasing in the months following the laparoscopic surgery I had in the summer of 2012 to diagnose and treat my endometriosis. But above all else, I was concerned about where the pain seemed to be located and what was triggering it. On top of a swelling abdomen and general GI issues, my vagina fucking hurt. I was struggling to wear pants, or underwear at all. I could barely stand to insert a tampon, and orgasming or feeling even slightly turned on was incomprehensible. The few times that I had attempted to be sexually active were disaster upon disaster and it was this, above all else, that really brought me to a breaking point.

For a long time I was in denial about what was happening in my body. In the months following my surgery, I was fully under the impression that my endometriosis was gone. I had undergone an ablation surgery—a surgery where doctors remove growths and scar tissue with a laser or attempt to destroy them with intense heat (which has since been proven ineffective)—and the doctor who performed the surgery had assured me, time and time again, that the pain I was now experiencing had nothing to do with my endometriosis. I thought I had come to terms with my diagnosis of endometriosis. But with reflection, I see now that I was able to "come to terms" with it because I *didn't understand it*. At all. I naively assumed that the endometriosis that had wrecked my teenage years was in my past and all I had to focus on was the present. And so much of that present was my inability to be sexual.

I've always considered myself to be a relatively sexual person. Maybe it's the Taurus in me, or maybe it's just the way I was built, but I enjoy being intimate. Learning this about myself, however, was extremely difficult in the midst of all the pain I was experiencing in the lower region of my body. Penetrative sex has always been impossible for me, though not for lack of trying. But prior to my laparoscopic surgery, I had experienced intimacy in other ways that had brought me great pleasure. It was a combination of desiring this pleasure and my desperate wish to feel a sense of normalcy that made me feel so fucking lost when I realized I was unable to experience pleasure in the way I expected anymore.

Having the ability to be sexually active might not be regarded as "normal" to everyone. But as a straight woman who was exclusively dating men in a world that is sex-filled, whether we acknowledge this or not, it was definitely *my* idea of normal. And at the time, sex to me was literally just the idea of a penis going into a vagina. This is probably because every man I had been sexual with up to this point had relied pretty much solely on penetration. It was also because painful sex and sex outside of a penis going into a vagina is rarely ever shown in the media, which is the basis for a lot of the world's knowledge about things that are otherwise considered a bit taboo for polite conversation, like sex. As the months progressed and the pain I felt when I orgasmed and when anything came in contact with my vulva in general became ever more present, my distress around this became less about the physical pain itself and more about the emotional pain I felt around it. I was ashamed. I felt like less of a person. I didn't feel desirable.

Even after I got some answers, it was this idea that I was broken in some way, or unable to give any partners everything that they deserved, that kept me in the dark clouds of depression for months after my initial diagnoses of what I now refer to as Vagina Problems.

I used to think the entire world was having penetrative sex but me. It seemed like everywhere I looked, people were referencing sex in some way. I couldn't go to the grocery store, to the movies, or to Starbucks without observing or overhearing some reference to sex. I couldn't even turn on the TV without seeing a commercial for a pill to "enhance your sex life." Sex was everywhere. It followed me, taunting me. I saw it on billboards and overheard it in conversations. I saw it referenced on drink menus at restaurants and heard about it during commercials on the radio. It was as if the whole world was sitting at one giant lunch table talking about their great sex lives and I was the outcast, walking by the table with my lunch tray in my hands, heading straight to the bathroom to eat my lunch alone in a stall. I was very much under the impression that every consenting adult was constantly having sex. And not only were they constantly having sex, they were having good sex. Great sex, even! There was no pausing to add a bunch more lube, or thirty minutes of foreplay to get someone's pelvic floor muscles used to the idea of being aroused without shooting pain. And there certainly wasn't room for people like me—people who couldn't have penetrative sex at all.

Prior to officially receiving my diagnoses of vulvodynia and vaginismus—involuntary contractions of the pelvic floor muscles and a throbbing ache in the vagina—at the Mayo Clinic, I didn't have much of a reference for what a well-rounded sex life could be. I had limited knowledge when it came to this, partly because sex had always been clouded with pain and was overall a relatively unpleasant and painful experience for me. My sexual escapades with my high school boyfriend and one or two men in college were really the only reference points I had at that time, and the reference wasn't too in-depth. Besides the fact that any other type of sex or intimacy beyond penis-in-vagina penetration is rarely ever portrayed in mainstream media, as I've mentioned, even that portrayal is also just a straight-up lie. Where is the lube? Where is the foreplay? Where is the dry humping? Where is the removal of glasses before sex? The peeing immediately after? The awkward squishing noises? The people who can't have sex because it's painful? The people who don't get off from penetration alone? The oral? The use of toys? The inability to orgasm at all sometimes? WHERE IS IT??

By the time I was in college in 2010, I mostly considered myself a virgin. I wasn't sure how else to describe someone who wanted to have sex, had tried, but couldn't due to unexplained pain. I actually used to joke with my friends about it. Like Regina in *Mean Girls*, who exclaimed, "I was half a virgin when I met him," I wore it like a badge of honor. *I'm, like, half a virgin,* I would tell my friends. They would laugh with me, thinking they were in on the joke. It was my way of explaining that my high school boyfriend and I *had* attempted penetration—but I left out the part where we had to stop after a thrust or two because it was so goddamn painful that it left me screaming, with tears pouring down my face.

Looking back now, I know my joking was a defense mechanism. I didn't know how to communicate the pain I was feeling in that part of my body. I wasn't even sure if what I was experiencing was out of the ordinary. For all I knew, perhaps everyone was experiencing this pain, but they were just better at handling it than me. And, after all, pain associated with sex wasn't a new concept to me. In many ways, I was taught to expect it. There are very few conversations regarding sex I can recall between classmates or friends when I was growing up that did not somehow include the mention of how painful it is for women their first time. I didn't just understand that sex *could* be painful for women who were new to it—I went into my first time *expecting* it to be painful. I just didn't expect it to be *that* painful.

I didn't want to try again after that for a long time. I avoided it completely. And since I had always been told sex would be painful the first couple of times, I assumed it was normal and never spoke of it to anyone. It wasn't like I was dying to bring it up in conversation, anyway. *Hey, remember when I said I was half a virgin? Haha, yeah. What I actually meant was that when I attempted to have sex I felt as if I were being ripped open from the inside out and a burning metal rod was searing my insides. The thought of attempting to do it again fills me with such fear and anxiety that I feel the urge to buy a real chastity belt. Is that what it felt like for you, too?*

As my college years continued and the topic of sex felt even more prevalent, I could feel myself sinking even more inward. I was embarrassed. I didn't know how to contribute to the conversations happening around me, and I wasn't even sure that someone like me was allowed to. I *wanted* to have sex. I had the urges. I found myself attracted to many men and yearned to lean in to their touch. But every time I felt myself doing this, my brain would force me to remember the pain associated with physical intimacy in the past. After that, my body would tense up and start to shake. I didn't know how to explain it or deal with it at all. So I made a joke out of it, kept calling myself half a virgin, and did my best to move on with my life—until I could no longer ignore the problem or pretend it wasn't happening.

* * *

Try as I might to forget the day I arrived in Rochester at the Mayo Clinic and went to my appointment with the gynecologist, I have yet to be successful. I started the trip feeling hopeful, sure that I would finally be given a solution to the pain I was experiencing. But I ended the trip feeling more helpless than ever before.

I was lying on my back with my feet in stirrups. I could feel my body starting to shake. The spot I was staring at on the ceiling was beginning to look like a pear. I focused harder on it, trying to distract myself from the discomfort. Pear, pear, pear. I could feel the sweat on the back of my neck slowly drip down my spine. My body was so tense. The deep breaths I kept attempting to take in an effort to unclench the muscles in my jaw were doing nothing.

I was surrounded by medical professionals. My mom was in the waiting room outside. I had wanted her there with me but had been too embarrassed to ask. I was wearing one of those hospital gowns and the entire lower half of my body was exposed. In the room with me were the famed director of gynecology at the Mayo Clinic and three medical students. All three of the medical students were men, and all three of them were close to my age. I did my best to remain dignified, but that's difficult to do when your legs are in stirrups and your vulva is exposed to three attractive medical students because you can't figure out why your vagina hurts so bad, especially during sex. It felt like an out-of-body experience. Even now, looking back on it, it's hard to place myself there.

Of course, I *was* there, and it was I who nodded in agreement when the main doctor told me she was going to poke my vulva with a Q-tip. "Do whatever you need to do," I said. Five seconds later I was gasping and screaming out in pain. "What are you DOING?" I yelled. She wheeled her stool back, looked at me, and held up the Q-tip. "I just gently placed this against your vulva." I didn't understand. "You have vulvodynia," she said. The room began going out of focus. I could see the edges blur. I didn't know what that word meant. She kept talking. I did my best to listen, but I could feel my heart beating faster and faster. As she continued talking, I was having trouble breathing. To this day, I cannot recount exactly what she said to me. But I remember the main points: *We do not have a definitive reason for this sort of vaginal pain, there is **no known cure**, and you need to go to physical therapy.* The physical therapy part was confusing to me. Why would I go to physical therapy for MY VAGINA?

As I was trying to process what she had said, I could feel the medical students looking at me. When I glanced up, I saw the concern and pity in their eyes. I felt like a child. I wanted to scream at all of them to please leave, to go away and never come back. I wanted them to turn away and not look at me for another second. I could feel myself breaking. The tears were coming faster. I could feel their eyes on me. I wanted to shove their faces away. I felt like an animal in a zoo. Like some poor runt of the litter that no one wanted to take home, but everyone wanted to stare at. I couldn't breathe, and I could barely make out the faces of the medical students through the tears that were now freely pouring out of my eyes. The main doctor got up to leave. "We'll give you some time to compose yourself." When I heard the door click and realized I was alone, I slid off the medical examining table, ripped off the medical gown, and lay naked on the floor.

I'm not sure how long I lay there on that cold, hard floor, letting the tears fall from my eyes down my chin to eventually pool on the floor beside me, but after a while I finally exhausted myself enough that, like Ariana Grande, I had no tears left to cry. I somehow found the strength to pick myself up and put my clothes back on. I didn't particularly want to leave, but I also sure as hell didn't want to stay.

As I was pulling my shirt back over my head, I caught a glimpse of myself in the mirror above the sink in the little exam room and almost didn't recognize myself. My eyes were red, swollen, bloodshot. I was covered in sweat; my lips were dry. My hair was frizzy and falling out of the braid I had delicately placed it in that morning in the hotel room across the street from the hospital. I looked frantic and felt even more so. I tried to compose myself. I knew I had to face my mom and try to recount what had just happened. I wanted to be strong, put on a brave face, and reassure her that everything was okay. Because, after all, wasn't it? I mean, I wasn't dying. I just might have vaginal pain for the rest of my life. What's the big deal, right?

When I had entered the room only an hour before, I was sure that I would get the answers I needed; what I never expected was an answer without a solution. Back then, I was still naive when it came to the medical system and its way of handling chronic illness and pain—especially pain associated with sex, and *especially* pain associated with women. I still believed that Western medicine held all the answers. Are you sick? There's a pill for that! Unexplained pain? There's an answer for that—and if you just do these things you'll feel better in no time! I wanted this to be true so badly. I *needed* it to be true. But of course, that wasn't how it happened.

Even so, this visit was instrumental in my life. It gave me the diagnoses I so desperately craved. The doctors gave me the vital information I needed about the pelvic floor, the way it can cease to function properly, and how pelvic floor physical therapy can help. I knew, at least in some ways, what I was up against. But what they didn't give me was the cure I so desperately sought. They weren't able to tell me if I would ever really be free of this. They couldn't tell me that I would be able to go on a date with someone in my future, fall for them, and be able to express that through intimacy without experiencing mind-boggling pain. They couldn't tell me that I would be able to live a life that didn't involve crying tears of shame as I removed my underwear in the bathroom stall at Olive Garden because it was agitating my vagina so much. At twenty-one years old, I was told that there was little to nothing that I could do about the pain I was experiencing that I very much felt was *ruining my life*. At twenty-one years old, I felt like my life was over.

I looked at the person staring back at me in the mirror once more before leaving the room. When she had entered the room, she was full of hope at the possibility of getting her life back. She had a light in her eyes. Now the light had been extinguished.

* * *

Most of what I was taught about sex was bullshit. Most of what the majority of us are taught about sex is bullshit, for that matter, but it's extra bullshit for women. One of my first memories on the subject of sex was in fifth grade, when they separated the boys and girls at school to go into different classrooms for "the talk." We spent a couple of hours, all of us girls jammed into one classroom, sitting cross-legged on the floor as we listened to our female teachers explain to us how periods worked. They showed us how to insert tampons on a stuffed doll. It all seemed relatively normal to me, and I had (thankfully) heard it all before. But when we took a break for recess and lunch, it became apparent that the boys in my class were learning something quite different. As I ran around from the swing set to the basketball court and back, I kept hearing the words "ejaculate" and "masturbate" from the boys in my class, followed by laughter. I had no idea what it meant. And I wasn't sure I ever wanted to learn. Did boys have a period, too? I wasn't sure. After lunch and recess we resumed our normal classwork and the subject wasn't brought up again until years later.

Fast forward to my high school years, my sophomore year specifically. I'm sitting in health class. By this point, I have a decent idea of what sex is, mostly because I rode the bus to school for most of my life, and the kids who sit in the back of the bus teach you some shit whether you want to learn it or not. My health teacher was explaining to us that we would be learning about sex today. A lot of people laughed, me included. We were fifteen-year-olds living in an extremely conservative area where the mention of sex was frowned upon, at best. We had no idea what we were in for. We all felt a little awkward and embarrassed. But it turned out, what we were going to be learning wasn't much. The teacher droned on in a monotone about how sex was something that happened when you got married in order to produce children. It was not supposed to happen in any other capacity. She continued, "It will feel good for the man and he will eventually ejaculate sperm, which is how babies are produced." I remember thinking that sex sounded gross. But looking back now, I also realize how damaging this type of messaging would be for years to come, when I started dealing with my problems with sexual pain and intimacy.

The messaging that I, and many other young girls, constantly received growing up is that sex was pleasurable *for the man*. It was also that sex = penetration. Period. Beyond the fact that this disregards the not-straight people living in this world, it's also incredibly damaging messaging to relay to young women. There was never a mention that sex could feel good for us, too. It wasn't even a factor.

Yes, I know we were only fifteen at the time, and you may not think pleasure or painful sex, or anything related to penises and vaginas, is appropriate to teach to fifteen-year-olds. But it's been shown time and time again that abstinence-only sex education does not work. We should be teaching teenagers about sex. Safe sex. Consensual sex. Painful sex and the disorders that may cause it. Maybe my sophomore year health class wasn't the perfect venue for this, but I wasn't learning it anywhere else, either. The very first time I found the courage to bring up painful sex to a doctor, I was *immediately* shamed for being sexually active. I was told it was wrong. It was something I should wait to do until marriage. That I was experiencing *mind-boggling pain* during intercourse wasn't concerning to my doctor. But me having sex outside of marriage was. I was nineteen years old. It took me years after that to ever bring it up again.

For so long, my understanding of sex was limited. What even was a female orgasm? Female masturbation? Oral sex? Sex for pleasure and not for babies? Intimacy? None of it existed to me. Sex was penetration and when, a couple of years after my sex ed talk in high school, I discovered that I couldn't have that without massive amounts of pain, I began to believe that I could not have sex at all.

You don't realize how many sexual references there are in the world until you no longer feel as if you can be a part of them in any way. Whereas before I might have been able to watch a soap opera in the middle of the day in between classes without feeling a hundred worms in my stomach, after I realized that I experienced pain with sex, suddenly that soap opera with the overdramatized sex scene made me feel like I had swallowed acid. Many things began to look different to me. And I began to feel different. I felt broken—as if something were wrong with me and the way my body did or did not function. I felt unwanted. And I no longer felt as if I were allowed to be a part of any conversation pertaining to sex. I stopped allowing myself to think about it or participate in conversations about it at all. I avoided dating. I changed the subject when my friends mentioned anything pertaining to sex. I no longer felt like I belonged, and I was trying desperately to find a way to be okay with this. Suddenly I was on the outside looking in. But despite how hard I tried to accept this, I had never felt so alone.

One of the feelings I recall most often in thinking about what it is like to live with any sort of Vagina Problems is how *isolating* it can be. Once I received my diagnoses of all my Vagina Problems, I thought I would have a better understanding of what I was up against and would therefore feel better about the situation. But what I didn't expect was just how fucking alone I felt. Despite knowing, on some level, that I couldn't possibly be the only person experiencing this type of pain every day and with intimacy, remembering this on my saddest days was difficult. I had no one to talk to about the burning I felt radiating throughout my vagina after wearing boy shorts underwear for an hour. I was embarrassed, ashamed, scared. And even if I had wanted to bring it up, I didn't know how.

The older I got, and the more I yearned to experiment with sex, the less I felt I was allowed to. It's difficult to explain, but although my pain was mostly emanating from my vagina, my whole body felt fragmented in one way or another. It wasn't just that I had pain with insertion or pain with climax, it was an overall feeling of rejection. I felt like my body was wrong in so many ways. If a man even considered spending time with me after they found out about my pain, I felt as if I owed them the world. Because of my lack of sexual knowledge and experience, I certainly wasn't suggesting to my partners that they go down on me or introduce toys into the mix. I couldn't see past my limitations to recognize the possibilities left behind.

It didn't take long before I began associating my entire self-worth with whether or not I could be sexually active. When it feels as if the whole damn world is having sex and you know that, despite your best efforts, you can't, it's nearly impossible to not have your self-esteem impacted in some way. I entered into unhealthy relationships simply because I so desperately craved intimacy, which I hoped might stop my internal belief that I was unworthy. Being with someone who treated me poorly somehow felt better than being alone, because alone I was simply reminded again and again that the way I worked was different and—in my mind—undesirable. I could tell myself until I was blue in the face that my inability to experience penetration did not make me any less desirable, but I never believed it. And I was the only one reassuring myself because I had no idea how to talk about this with anyone else, and I was so embarrassed I couldn't even try.

I can really only recall a few times over the years when I attempted to open up to my doctors about the pain I experienced during sex. But I was always told the same shit: *Just push through the pain. Drink wine beforehand to get yourself to "relax." Use lube. Try a different position.* Or, my personal favorite: *You seem to be imagining this pain.* And when I tried to bring my issues up during conversation with anyone—a doctor or a friend—the subject was always left hanging in the air like a silent-but-deadly fart that you didn't think anyone would notice but that everyone definitely noticed, and now no one knows what to say. This was partly because I was never sure how to bring up the topic and partly because it's not a subject people are accustomed to discussing. *Anyone had any good mind-boggling pain during sex lately? Anyone run crying and screaming from the bedroom of a guy on the football team after he got a half inch of his dick inside you? No? Oh. Cool.*

I would try desperately, every so often, to fit in and be a part of my friends' conversations—"Oh yeah, I might sleep with Tom tonight"—while deep down, my insides were squirming at the thought. My whole life began to feel like one giant lie. I was living with an enormous secret. My Vagina Problems followed me everywhere I went, like a big, angry cloud casting a shadow over everything I did, invisible to everyone but me. The more I tried to ignore the cloud, the bigger it became. It felt easier to pretend that I was getting to second and third base with various men in college than it did to try to explain that a man even giving me a compliment sent me into such a panicked state that I would have to lie on my dorm room bed for hours, reminding myself how to breathe.

That is what needs to be understood about Vagina Problems: It isn't just the physical pain of not being able to have anything inserted into my vagina, or a shooting ache in my pelvis any-time I feel aroused—it is an entire psychological state where I began to associate absolutely everything related to sex or inti-macy of any kind with mind-boggling pain. It was no longer just a man touching the small of my back, it was a man trying to initiate intimacy, and all I could envision was my own phys-ical pain and his disappointed and annoyed face when I could not perform the way I thought I was supposed to.

My Vagina Problems were taking over my life. And I felt powerless to stop them. But instead of acknowledging this, I did my best to pretend it wasn't happening. I thought that maybe if I refused to acknowledge the discomfort, it would eventually go away. If I denied it enough, maybe I could convince myself it wasn't happening. The lies I spun about the life I *wished* I was having got out of control. A sense of normalcy, or just the ability to kiss a man without so much dread that I would end up on my bathroom floor puking, was something I so desperately craved, I could almost taste it. Eventually I was not only lying to my friends and pretending that I was fine, having sexual encounters, and living a normal twentysomething-year-old's life—I was also lying to myself. I believed that if I kept telling myself I was fine with it, that the discomfort was all in my head, eventually I would be.

I was wrong.

* * *

Despite being given a diagnosis for my pain, which in and of itself implied that other people had experienced it before, I still often felt that I was the only person with the problem. But about a year after my initial diagnoses of vulvodynia and vaginismus, my pelvic floor physical therapist and I started a support group for women in the Indianapolis area who were experiencing painful sex. It was then I realized I wasn't alone. It's almost laughable to think about now—to think that I actually believed that pain associated with sex was not relatively common. But why would I believe any different when every message I was receiving was the opposite? Why would any of us? The message we all received was the same: sex, sex, sex, and more sex. Everyone seemed to be having it. Everyone, I thought, but me.

Meeting other women with the same problem was earth-shattering for me. But most of the women in the group were married and much older than I was at the time. They had already gone through their dating days. They had experienced their twenties without their Vagina Problems. While it didn't make their pain any less, it did mean that I still felt alone in some ways. However, that group gave me the courage to finally acknowledge my Vagina Problems and the pain I was experiencing every day. Even if it was just to myself at first. I was twenty-two years old but felt decades older. I was barely out of college and had never felt more lost. I'm not even sure I realized what I was doing at first. It all just came spilling out of me. I started slowly. I told my closest friend, through tears, that dating was going to be really hard for me for the foresee-able future. Then, a couple of weeks later, I told a man that I was acquaintances with through Skype messaging. Then, I told another man—this time via Facebook messenger. I found myself repeatedly fighting the urge to reach out to men spe-cifically to confide to them about this part of my life. But I desperately wanted a man to tell me that he was okay with my Vagina Problems.

Things also started to change for me after I wrote an essay for Buzzfeed.com about how sex was painful for me in April of 2014—just three months after I started my job at the company. Up to that point, fewer than five people in my life knew about the pain I had been experiencing. Prior to this, the cloud of my Big Secret had felt heavier and heavier; now I could no longer keep the secret inside of me. I could not find my voice to speak about it out loud, so I wrote about it instead. While a part of me knew that it would be published on a website that people—everyone I had ever known, including, potentially, my high school math teacher—could see and read, that didn't register. I just wanted to be free of the secret that had been weighing so heavily on me for so long. I wanted it out of me. I felt like I was being eaten alive.

After my essay was published, I felt as if a weight had been lifted from my shoulders. I felt as if I could breathe again. I didn't know it at the time, but writing that essay was one of the best things I've ever done for myself, in part because it was healing to finally talk about the agony I had been experiencing for so long, and in part because that essay gave me what I didn't know I so desperately needed: the knowledge that I was far from being alone.

Messages from people all over the world came pouring into my inbox, slowly but surely, all telling me the same thing: You are not alone. Suddenly, the weight of living with Vagina Problems didn't feel quite as heavy anymore. My vagina still hurt, of course, but knowing that it was hurting in conjunction with other people's vaginas made the mental aspect of it all hurt a little less.

* * *

Part of the reason I chose to write this book is because it is what I wish I had when I was nineteen years old and starting to really understand the pain I was feeling—and understand that it wasn't going away. I so desperately wish that I had had someone in my life to tell me that sex was much more than a penis in a vagina. I wish I had been privy to the fact that many women don't even climax from penetration alone. I wish I had known that what I was experiencing was not uncommon or rare, and that I was certainly not alone. I wish I had known that it wasn't my fault, and that I had done nothing to cause it. I wish I had known that while there may not be a definitive cure, there are things I can do to help. I yearn for nineteen-year-old Lara to know that you can have sex and be intimate in a thousand different ways, and that zero of those ways determine your worth in any relationship. I also wish nineteen-year-old Lara had known that it was okay to be upset about this. It was okay to be angry and feel slighted and be sad and mourn for the life she thought she was going to have but never did. Lara, at nineteen years old, didn't know these things. But I know them now. I want this book to be a friend to people. I want you to know that no matter how alone you may feel—you are not alone. Not really. I want you to know that your feelings, all of them, are valid.

In the time since I began to publicly and privately talk about the pain I have experienced since my teenage years, I have had many realizations. I now know that I am not alone in this—not even close. I have experienced the highest of highs and the lowest of lows. I have made such progress, and I have reverted to the beginning. I have learned a lot about myself, about the medical community, and about women's health care. I have tried countless alternative treatments and experienced a thousand different side effects from various drugs. I have shed many tears. I've dated, had casual sex, been in relationships. I've orgasmed without much pain—and I've orgasmed and then been in so much pain that I could not leave the bed. I have picked up the broken pieces of myself in many hospital exam rooms and put myself back together again. I am not free of my Vagina Problems, almost seven years to the day from my original diagnosis. I'm not sure I will ever really be free of them. But these days, I don't hold so tightly to the idea of getting rid of them. These days, I see them as a part of me—for better or worse. I do not believe in the idea that going through pain like this is something to be grateful for. That it somehow makes me a stronger person, or more empathetic. I am not grateful for my pain. But I am grateful for the person I have become in spite of it.

2

"My Vagina Just Hurts a Lot" and How to Explain What the Hell Else Is Actually Going On

Endometriosis. Vulvodynia. Vaginismus. Pelvic Floor Dysfunction. Vulvar Vestibulitis. Interstitial Cystitis. Dyspareunia. Premenstrual dysphoric disorder. Adenomyosis. Dysmenorrhea. Ovarian Cysts. Fibrocystic breasts. These are just some of the terms that have been thrown my way over the last decade as an explanation for the war raging inside my body. I used to keep better track. I would research each of them for hours on end, taking notes in a notebook I bought at Target because it had sunflowers on the cover. I would pore over whatever information I could get my hands on and do my best to keep track of every "do" or "don't" I found related to each new ailment I was presented with. I bought a pack of pens at Target, too. They were colorful and bright, and I would alternate the colors I wrote with. The dos were written in a bright green, my favorite color, while the don'ts were sketched in purple . . . a color I never really cared for much.

I would itemize each list and underline and star any

triggers that seemed to correlate among ailments. Eventually, it got too hard to keep track. One message board would tell me to never touch turmeric because of my bladder pain, yet another would tell me that I should be ingesting it every day to help with the inflammation endometriosis caused in my body. One message board would suggest a completely plant-based diet, but when I actually ate that way, my abdomen would swell so suddenly and swiftly that I would have to lie down within thirty minutes, scorching that same spot on my stomach with a heating pad for hours after.

Eventually, I had to stop poring over my lists of dos and don'ts and hide them away on a high shelf in the corner of my closet behind a suitcase to stop obsessing over them. It's not that I didn't want to do my best to follow the guidelines that others had tirelessly tried and tested over the years in an effort to help others. I did. But at some point, during the time I was sleeping every night on my back with my legs propped up because a blog told me to and drinking celery juice on an empty stomach every morning while meticulously keeping track of every single thing I did, I forgot how to live.

It's often challenging to explain the varieties of pain that come with my Vagina Problems—and the way in which they are all connected, yet different. I used to do my best to explain to people my different diagnoses and how they contribute to the pain I feel. But it doesn't make much sense to most people. And why would it? Most of the time it barely makes sense to me, the person living with it.

I could tell you, for example, that endometriosis is when tissue that is similar to the uterine lining is found on other organs. But what does that really mean? Even to me, a person with tissue similar to the uterine lining actively being found on other organs, it doesn't mean much. In addition, up until a few years ago, most people had never even heard of endometriosis at all. Tissue being found on other organs and some random word—"endometriosis"—don't sound painful. But telling you that I sometimes wish for death as an alternative to the pain . . . that feels like a more accurate description.

I could then tell you that vulvodynia is chronic vulvar pain with no known cause that is often identifiable by a "Q-tip test," where a doctor will simply touch the vulva with a Q-tip to see where it's painful. But again, what does that mean? It feels more accurate to tell you that if I wear high-waisted skinny jeans, my vagina will be burning so fiercely by lunchtime that I will then spend the entire evening alternating between rubbing coconut oil on my vulva and pressing an ice pack against it.

And then I could tell you that vaginismus is involuntary muscle spasms of the pelvic floor, making the insertion of things (whether that be a penis, a crystal dildo, or a tampon) nearly impossible. But again, it feels more accurate to tell you that a penis attempting to go inside my vagina feels as if I am being ripped open with a giant chainsaw covered in acid.

Sometimes I do have the urge to tell people these things. Sometimes I want to say, "My periods are so painful because of my endometriosis that I am often paralyzed for forty-eight hours or more per month." But people don't always react well to honesty like that. It can make them uncomfortable. And sometimes I just don't have the energy or patience to explain things. Most people in my life assume that endometriosis is the only cause of all my pain—the painful sex, the vaginal burning, the inability to drink carbonated beverages without a swelling, burning bladder—all of it. And while I do believe endometriosis may be the catalyst for many of my issues, it is not the only problem going on here. There are around ten so far, and those are just the ones I can remember off the top of my head.

Sometimes I think of my illnesses as a night out filled with decisions you later regret. The endometriosis is the shots of cheap vodka you kick back at your friend's apartment before getting in the Uber. That is the beginning of it all. Perhaps if you had not indulged in that cheap vodka at the beginning of the night you would not end up with your head in the toilet puking your guts out by 11 P.M. But who knows? The vulvo-dynia and vaginismus are the two beers you drink at the bar as soon as you get there because they cost two dollars and what the hell? You're already mixing alcohol, but you're hav-ing fuuuuun. It's cheap. Who cares? What could go wrong? The interstitial cystitis is the shot of tequila someone buys you because they "love your energy." The PMDD, cystic breasts, and ovarian cysts are the Jack and Coke you down after you hear your favorite Lizzo song come on. And the rest—well, it's kind of a blur after that, isn't it?

When I made the decision to be open about the pain I was experiencing, I wanted to find a way to make talking about it easier on myself. I didn't want to have to explain each of my symptoms to people every single time my illnesses were brought up in conversation, but I also didn't want to give some textbook-sounding definition and watch as their eyes glazed over. And I didn't want to feel like I had to avoid talking about something that impacts my life in no small way every single day. More than all of this, though, I had the desire to take back ownership. It is not surprising that I often feel as if I do not have control over my own life because of the illnesses I live with. They have dictated so many things, so many moments. And I've never gotten a say in any of it. The one thing I do have a say in, though, is how I react to it. It was up to me to decide how I wanted to present my pain and illnesses and all the shit that comes with them to the world. And in doing that, I wanted it to feel like the way the discussion went was completely my choice. I wanted to destigmatize the conversation around vaginas and period pain, and I wanted to make it more relatable. So Vagina Problems was born.

"I have Vagina Problems." I think the first time I ever said it was in the 2014 article I published on Buzzfeed.com. It was tangentially related to living with my illnesses, and I was trying to figure out whether or not I should type out every single diagnosis I had been given thus far with an explainer for each. It's a lot of emotional labor to go into every single thing, and I'm also not a lab rat, so sometimes I avoid going into too much detail. Partly because it's exhausting and partly because when I have done that in the past, I almost always got a bunch of "doctors" telling me the ways in which I was wrong. I made the decision not to type out every single diagnosis, but I still needed a way to acknowledge them in case any readers had pelvic pain and problems with their own vaginas. It came out naturally—my vagina (and the surrounding areas) had a lot of problems. So I typed it. No one really knows what "vulvodynia" means anyway, unless you have it. (And even when you have it, you still might not know because if you've learned anything thus far reading this book, I hope it's that the medical system fails those of us with Vagina Problems every single day.)

I needed something to express what was going on in my body that didn't undermine the pain I was experiencing but that also wasn't a twelve-hundred-word essay about every diagnosis I'd been given and the symptoms associated with it. "Vagina Problems" felt like the perfect description at the time. Although my pain is by no means isolated in my vagina, it often feels like the place where it all started. Some of the first pain I recall having was when I was bleeding during my period. From there, it began to flow throughout my entire abdomen and up my spine until it eventually infiltrated my entire body. But it started there.

Sometimes, when I'm high, I think about the term Vagina Problems and the way I have used it to describe something that has been so debilitating. I created a simple term that made me sort of laugh to think about. I can see that I wanted to take ownership back. I wanted to be in charge of how I presented this information to the world—and how they would feel about it when I did. I learned a long time ago that if I tried to divulge my various diagnoses and their symptoms, people's eyes would glaze over. The information didn't mean much to anyone who wasn't living with the problems. And it especially didn't mean much when I didn't feel comfortable saying, "Yeah my vagina burned so badly today that I literally can't stand to wear underwear and I just used your bathroom five minutes ago to rub coconut oil all over my vulva. Thanks, by the way!"

Saying things like that is taboo. It's uncomfortable. I wasn't ready to be completely honest about my vagina yet, and the world wasn't ready for that either. But I was getting there. I wanted the world to know that my pain was related to my vagina. Thus, Vagina Problems was born. It was a cutesy name. It was my way of taking this pain and saying, "Whatever. I'm here. I have it. It sucks. Let's talk about it." Because as much as I want Vagina Problems to be palatable so that we can talk about them, I also want to really talk about them. I want all these words, the different diagnoses for Vagina Problems, to be so recognizable one day that I can walk into a store, say, "I have vulvodynia," and immediately be directed to the area of the store with dresses that don't require underwear and pants that don't murder my vagina.

These terms, the many different ones I've been given over the years, are related. They are not uncommon. They are debilitating, awful, and all-consuming. So why are they still so unknown? Why in the world is it so hard to get a diagnosis? And why is it that when we finally manage to get a diagnosis, it's so damn hard to get treated?

I am forever grateful to the doctor I saw at the Mayo Clinic who not only gave me a diagnosis of pelvic floor dysfunction and related conditions, but told me to see a pelvic floor physical therapist. I had seen countless doctors for these issues prior to this appointment and not one of them had ever even mentioned pelvic floor physical therapy as an option. Outside of those doctors, I myself had never heard of this area of medicine before. I had no fucking idea that you could go to physical therapy for your vagina. And I am not alone. I still receive messages almost every day from people around the globe who were shocked to learn about pelvic floor physical therapy when I mentioned it online.

But why? If you think in terms of just how common these conditions are, and then think about the number of people who deliver babies every month—which, by the way, can wreak havoc on your pelvic floor—it seems completely asinine that pelvic floor physical therapy is still this unheard of. In my opinion, every person with a vulva/vagina/uterus should see a pelvic floor physical therapist at some point in their life. Not only for issues like mine, but because the pelvic floor deals with A LOT OF FUCKING SHIT. We hold emotions there. We store trauma. We give birth to babies and go through countless menstrual cycles. Yet some of the most common treatments for pelvic pain—that is, when it is actually diagnosed and taken seriously—are invasive procedures or dangerous prescription drugs that come with so many side effects, you can't tell if what you're experiencing is from your pelvic pain or from the medicine.

I am not a doctor. I am not a researcher. I did not go to grad school. I barely graduated from college. I struggle to comprehend basic medical studies. I mispronounced the word "anatomy" until last year. But I am confident in saying that I know more about the pelvic floor—and how to treat pelvic pain— than 90 percent of the doctors I have seen in my lifetime. And I've seen a lot of doctors. It's not that I am spending my free time going to the library and reading everything about pelvic pain that I can get my hands on. I'm not. When would I find the time amid watching 90 *Day Fiancé* reruns and every single show on the Bravo network? But I am living with it. And I have lived with pelvic pain for more than a decade now. And because I was given no viable solutions for this pain for most of this time, I had to find my own. I had to become my own doctor, my own advocate, my own research assistant.

I don't expect doctors to know everything I know about pelvic pain at this point. I understand it's unrealistic. Naturally someone living with this pain would have a better understanding of it than someone who is not. But I expect doctors to know *something* about it. I expect them to be able to offer more than "Sex is painful sometimes" as a response to mind-boggling vaginal pain.

Last summer I went to San Diego for a weekend. I was going to see an old friend from college whom I had always wanted to make out with and never got the chance. We went to a horse race as soon as I arrived and met up with a bunch of his friends. One of these friends was in med school. I started asking him about his experience. He mentioned that he was in a class specifically dedicated to women's health. I immediately asked him if they had learned about endometriosis, since it had become more well known and talked about in recent years. He told me they had. I asked him what they had learned. He said, "Well, it's a condition that makes women's periods pretty painful." I waited, thinking he would say more. He did not. My mouth dropped open. "Is that all you learned?" I asked. "That's the gist of it," he said. I wish I had been more shocked. But mostly, I expected it. I *wish* endometriosis were just a painful period. I think we all do.

Moments like this used to completely overwhelm me and leave me feeling dejected. I would be so angry and so disappointed that I could hardly stand it every time a medical professional showed that kind of ignorance when it came to my Vagina Problems. It made me want to give up. It made me ask myself, *WHAT IS THE FUCKING POINT?* These days, when things like this happen, I still get angry. But I also find a way to get even. Don't worry, I'm not, like, egging doctors' houses or anything. At least not yet. But I am fighting back, in my own way. I am talking about my vagina, and all its problems, whenever the hell I want to. I am acknowledging that sex is painful for me while also allowing myself to declare that I still deserve to orgasm. I am standing up and leaving doctors' offices when I feel they are not giving me adequate care. I am reminding them that *they* work for *me*. I am demanding better care. And I am demanding to be listened to. When a medical professional shows me that they still have no fucking clue how to talk about or treat Vagina Problems, it fuels me. When I leave their office, the rage I feel inside pushes me to continue living with this, advocating for it, talking about it, and demanding the attention it deserves.

The idea that something can be this widespread, chronic,

and painful, and still be so misunderstood is, honestly, shocking. It's estimated that one in ten women have pain during penetration. Almost two hundred million people around the world live with endometriosis, which is also one in ten women. And pelvic pain in general is not uncommon. Not by a long shot. Yet the treatment options available for any of these would make you think it was. People assume that something this common would surely have more options. It can't possibly be this misunderstood, with so few treatment routes. But it is. So the notion becomes that you *must* be able to regulate the pain somehow, you just aren't trying hard enough!

Sadly, doctors reinforced this idea in me for years. It was never a question of whether the medical community had advanced far enough to help me (and others like me) yet—it was just my fault. Period. I was either too stressed out or too depressed. I was anxious. I needed intense therapy. I wanted attention. Everybody had pain, I just wasn't good at dealing with it. Periods were just *supposed* to be painful. I needed to drink wine, relax. I was eating the wrong things according to one doctor, and eating too much according to another. I needed to eat small meals throughout the day and never drink cold or hot beverages, said one, while another said if I followed a keto-like diet I would be "symptom-free" in mere weeks. If I'd listened to one doctor, I would have had a total hysterectomy at age twenty-two. If I'd listened to another, I would have gotten pregnant in an attempt to "cure" my endometriosis. If the cause for my pain wasn't related to my diet according to doctors, or to the idea that I was just a Sad Gurl imagining it all, it was simply that I wasn't taking the right medicine. Never mind that I was recommended five wildly different prescriptions by five different doctors, somehow it was still my fault. And after a while, it became hard to believe anything else.

The "What If" game will consume you if you let it. I've spent hours, weeks, likely *months* of my life keeping track of every single thing I did or every single thing I put in my body. I would make list after list after list, jotting down things like the oat milk I consumed with my breakfast that morning—exactly twelve ounces—in an effort to pinpoint the exact cause of the ache in my abdomen I felt later in the day. I would keep track of every time I moved out of bed, and the way in which my feet hit the ground. I noted what sort of incline I was walking on, and what kind of shoes I was wearing at the time. I sifted through my underwear drawer and sorted them into categories—"might hurt my vagina," "will definitely hurt my vagina," and "maybe safe to wear but honestly unsure because even though I wore them nine times without pain, one time I was in pain and I can't tell if there's a correlation." After a while, the meticulous lists and obsession over every move I made stopped being helpful and started to become downright hurtful. I became my own enemy.

Sure, I pinpointed some triggers. For example, I noticed that consuming any type of soy triggers a pain flare in me that will last for days. I also noticed that almond milk is a no-go, and that my fresh-pressed juice that I so love in the mornings needs to have ginger added to it. I became very aware that certain brands of yoga pants did more harm to my body than good, and that walking at an incline without stretching my hip flexors out afterward definitely wasn't something I should ever do.

But I also began to berate myself. If I enjoyed a cookie at an office get-together with coworkers, I would spend hours afterward staring at my list and telling myself that it had to be my fault that I was in pain. I could not leave the house without finding a way in which my pain was my fault. I was walking wrong. I wore the wrong kind of underwear. I didn't stretch enough. I needed to go to yoga more. This self-blame became toxic. I could no longer pretend it was helpful. And what was becoming increasingly clear above all else was that I could do absolutely everything right—I could avoid soy, never touch almond milk, not eat an ounce of sugar or ever let caffeine touch my lips, walk slowly and in the right shoes while doing my stretches afterward—and I would still be in pain. And when I realized that, I lost my ability to care as much about the lists . . . or anything at all. Realizing that I could seemingly do absolutely everything right and still be in pain was a very hard pill to swallow.

In some ways, this realization allowed me to breathe again. I felt a sense of relief. The heavy weight of blame I had shouldered for so many years suddenly felt a bit lighter. But in other ways, the realization brought on a whole new bout of depression and anxiety that I wasn't equipped to deal with. What do you do about illnesses and pain that seemingly have no cause? How do you deal with being in massive amounts of pain—so much that breathing often feels difficult—when you can't figure out what the hell you did to cause it? How do you live? How do you go anywhere knowing that your body can rebel at any moment and you will be given no warning or reason? It would be easier if I had something to blame.

In many, many ways, blaming myself felt easier. It would be simpler to say, "I ate sugar and now I am in pain" than "I have no idea why I am in pain today, I have not consumed anything, I have not even left bed yet." Deep down I am aware that there *is* a reason for my pain—I have a disease. But that reasoning doesn't hold up when you've been stuck in bed for a week and all you've done is drink water and eat saltine crackers. I want a real reason for this pain—outside of "you have a disease"—because it feels like if I had a reason, then maybe I could find some sort of solution. If someone told me that eating sugar was causing it and that if I stopped doing that indefinitely, the disease would go away, I would do that. But that's not how Vagina Problems work. And once I figured that out, I had to figure out how the hell they *did* work, and how I was going to find a way to work with them.

Sometimes it seems as if my body is against me. I often describe these illnesses as feeling as if I am at war with my own body. And that is truly what it feels like. I feel as if I am punished or taken to battle constantly, for the littlest of things. And sometimes for nothing at all. But when it came down to it, finding a way to work with my Vagina Problems meant also finding a way to work with my body. I needed to find a way to accept the pain it put me through while also being able to accept that it was **not to punish me.** No matter how much it felt that way. My body is—and always has been—doing the best it can. It's been through hell and back and it is still here, doing its best, just like I am. Being on my own side has been crucial in finding a way to coexist with my Vagina Problems. Berating myself, blaming myself, and denying myself things simply because I felt as if all this pain was my fault has never made me feel any better. It's only made me feel worse. Being mad at my own body for something it has no control over only succeeded in making everything hurt even more.

If I am going to live with these Vagina Problems—and I am because I have been given no choice in the matter—then I am going to do it in a way that still feels like living. I don't want to be at war with my body and keep constantly checking my list of dos and don'ts. But I also don't want to go off the rails and do things that I know only make my pain worse. So I have done my best to find a way to exist somewhere in the middle. It's a place where I do my best to eat plant-based, low-sugar, gluten-free, and dairy-free foods while also eating a fucking cookie with my coworkers during happy hour if I want to. But it's not just eating the cookie. It's eating the cookie and knowing that the cookie is not the reason for my pain. It is allowing myself to live and acknowledging that my body is doing the best it can. It is hearing that voice inside my head that says, "You probably wouldn't be in pain if you didn't eat that cookie," and telling it to shut the fuck up. Because the truth is, I'd still be in pain. But I'd be in pain without experiencing the pleasure of eating a cookie. And that's not the kind of life I want to have.

3

This Is Endometriosis

You are on the bathroom floor. You are covered in sweat. You feel both as if you are running a fever and as if you are standing outside in twelve-degree weather without a coat on. Your body is shaking. You have just finished throwing up in your toilet but can't find the strength to lift your hand to your mouth to wipe the residue off your lips. Your head hurts from hitting it on the floor after you collapsed backward once your body was done forcing the pure stomach acid—because you haven't eaten in hours—out of your system. The floor is uncomfortable, and it's as if you can feel the hardness in every part of your body. But you prefer the uncomfortable feeling of the floor digging into your spine over the searing pain you feel in your abdomen. There's so much pressure on your uterus you feel like it might fall out of your vagina. It feels like you might give birth—but you know you're not pregnant. You can feel your heart racing; you're starting to panic. The pain is bad, it's really bad, and if history counts for anything, you know it's not going to get better anytime soon. It feels as if your insides are ripping apart. You wonder if stabbing yourself in the stomach would be less painful. You fantasize about grabbing the knife from your kitchen and plunging it in, if only to stop the other pain you are feeling for a little bit.

You have the brief thought that you should find your phone and try to call for help, but then the pain seizes you again and you can't imagine lifting a finger, let alone your whole body, to grab your phone. You think about screaming out and wonder if a neighbor would hear you and call 911. But then you realize you're not sure you'll be able to survive the time between now and when the ambulance would arrive. And even when you try to muster a scream, all that comes out is a faint moan of pain. You wonder if this is going to be the one that kills you. You wonder how you've ever made it out alive before. Your breathing accelerates more. In fact, you feel as if you can no longer breathe at all. You start losing feeling in your fingers and your toes. Then you feel that numbing sensation spreading all over your body—as if a foreign object is taking control of every nerve in your body, one by one. It's not freedom from the pain—you wish—but more of a tightening sensation, making it so you can no longer writhe around on the floor in an effort to distract yourself from the tearing apart of your insides. You tell yourself that it is going to pass. It always has. You tell yourself over and over and over again that you've been through this before. *It will pass. It will pass. It will pass.* You force yourself to repeat your own name back to yourself in an effort to remember that you are still alive, still breathing. The pain intensifies, and you stop trying to say your name and stop telling yourself that it will pass. You stop being able to communicate with yourself at all. There is no past, present, or future. There is no sense of time, or sense of reality. There is only the pain. The pain strips you of your identity, your body, and your life. It leaves you with nothing but the burning fire and stabbing sensation in your abdomen that is now spreading throughout your body.

The pain is so intense that it takes over every part of you. There is nothing in your brain anymore. Only pain. You briefly recall hearing yourself scream. You think you feel your dog licking your toes, but you're no longer sure you even have a dog. You're doing your best to hang on to reality, but reality is where the pain is. You beg and plead with the universe, the higher powers, whatever is out there, to please just make it stop. You fantasize about throwing yourself at the toilet and hitting your head so hard that you lose consciousness and can no longer feel anything at all. You try to move but all you can do is moan in pain. You feel the pain in your stomach and lower back swell again, and you flail your body sideways into the fetal position. You use your hands to press so hard against your stomach you fear you might throw up again, but any distraction from the pain is welcome. Your arms give out. You feel your body start to seize. Then everything fades to black, and you can no longer see or feel anything at all.

* * *

Waking up after an attack, I can't remember where I am. When reality starts to set in and I remember why I am on the ground, I feel panic start to rise in my chest once more. *Fuck, is it going to come back? Is it still here?* Before even allowing myself to take a full breath, I lie as still as I can and try to feel for any signs of the pain beginning to rile itself up again. My entire body hurts. But not like it did before. Nothing like that. It feels as if I am covered in bruises. My eyes struggle to focus, and I feel nauseous. My skin feels sticky. I can smell vomit, and I can feel the tears mixed with sweat plastering my hair to my forehead.

I try to find the strength to roll over and crawl to my bedroom in search of my phone. I have no idea what time it is or how long I've been out. Is it even the same day? As I start to roll over, I see my dog lying on the floor beside me. When she sees me moving, her tail starts wagging. Tears begin pouring out of my eyes. My dog, Pepper, is always nearby during my attacks these days, even when I don't know it. I want to pet her, to thank her for being there with me, but I don't have the energy. I feel guilty. The guilt starts to overwhelm me until I feel as if my chest might cave in on itself. I try to stay focused.

I get myself up on my forearms and take a few moments to steady my breathing. Everything is spinning. A few moments pass, and I am able to sit up. Though I know, based on past experience, that the attack is probably gone for the time being, my body is terrified with every move it makes. I half crawl, half walk to my bedroom and see my phone on the floor next to my bed. I grab it. It is 3:37 P.M. The last text I sent was at 9:43 A.M. It said, "It hurts so bad." I sent it to my friend Pablo. I always text him during really bad flares, in part because it's impossible not to want to talk about it when the pain is overtaking me, and in part because I want someone to know that if I don't answer for several hours, I likely need help. He had responded within a few minutes, but I never got the chance to open his message before the pain overpowered my ability to text. I open it now. It says, "It will pass. It always does. Just hang on as best you can until then." He had texted twice more after that, since I hadn't responded. One says, "Is it still bad?" The other says, "If you don't respond soon I am going to come over." It has only been a few hours—but it felt like a few years. I want to shower, to wash the stickiness and the memory of the last five or so hours of my life away. But I don't have the energy. I crawl into bed and feel my body sink into the mattress. I have the thought that I need to take Pepper outside so that she can go to the bathroom. But I am so tired. So, so tired. I lie in bed and try to close my eyes.

I want to sleep, but my mind forces me to think about what just happened. I think about how many times this has happened to me now. I can feel the exhaustion deep in my bones. As reality starts setting in and I recall what my body just went through, it feels as if a dark cloud is invading my brain, casting a giant shadow over any hope or optimism I might've had about living with these illnesses. I try to stop it. I tell myself not to go there. I try to remind myself of the reasons I have to be alive . . . of the things in my life that still feel worth living for.

But I have no fight left in me anymore. I ask myself how I am going to continue being able to live alone—or live at all. I wonder how I am ever going to be able to get out of bed again. I wonder, for a brief second, if Pepper will pee on my new cream-colored rug from Target because I am unable to take her outside. Then I wonder how I will be able to keep Pepper if I continue to have days where I cannot physically move. I feel guilty and start to wonder if I did something wrong. *Did I eat the wrong things? Is it because I had too much sugar this month? Was it that glass of prosecco? I need to go to acupuncture more. I haven't been to physical therapy in weeks. Why can't I be better about this shit? Why can't I just fucking take care of myself? When will I ever learn?*

Truthfully, it's not my fault that I'm in pain. But when you have no real reason for the pain, no one else to blame, and at least five years' worth of doctors suggesting that the pain is somehow your fault, you blame yourself anyway. These thoughts continue to swirl around in my brain until my chest becomes tighter and tighter and I eventually fall into a sleep-like state. I am neither unconscious nor conscious, but somewhere in between. Part of me is scared of falling asleep. I'm scared to give in to my exhaustion and drift off after an attack because part of me wonders if I'll ever wake up again—if my body will even bother to keep fighting. But another part of me is scared of staying awake and continuing to think because I fear that the longer I think about what just happened, the longer I will question whether I even want to keep fighting at all. If I fall asleep now, will I want to wake up again? Sometimes physically getting out of bed is only part of my battle; I have to mentally get myself out of bed, too. And after an attack, mentally getting up and choosing to continue fighting is the hardest part.

* * *

Even as I sit here typing this, the attack I experienced less than a week ago still somehow feels like a dream. I was there, I remember it happening, but the memory of it feels far away, as if someone else experienced it while I watched it unfold. I know that the pain was there, and I can still feel the exhaustion in my bones after living through it. But I can't remember exactly how it felt. After a decade of living with endometriosis, it feels more accurate to describe it not as just a chronic illness, but as a recurring nightmare—one I desperately wish I could wake from.

People have often asked me to describe endometriosis pain to them. And despite living with it for so long, I still struggle to find the words sometimes. There are, of course, different kinds of endometriosis pain. There are the days when it hurts just enough to drive you crazy but not enough to make you stay in bed—like a tiny pebble in your shoe all day that, no matter how hard you shake your shoe, simply won't come free. Then there are the days when you don't even realize you're hurting because you're so accustomed to the ache, and it's only after you've screamed at someone for cutting you off in traffic and then immediately started crying that you realize, *Oh, yeah, I'm in pain today.*

But there's also the pain that makes living with something like endometriosis impossible to wrap my mind around, regardless of how many years I've spent dealing with it. It's this pain that completely overtakes you. The attack. That's what it feels like—a disease attacking every inch of my body and rendering me completely helpless. These are the scariest days for me. They are the days I think about every time I feel the familiar ache in my abdomen or lower back and wonder how bad it will get this time. *Will I be able to get up? Will I be able to form thoughts at all? What if it happens while I'm driving? Or in Target? Would I even be able to get out of bed and leave my house if it caught on fire while I was in this amount of pain? What if I pass out from the pain and hit my head on the side of the counter and never wake up again?*

I think about these days before I go to sleep at night, and whenever I think about my future. These days haunt me, following me wherever I go. They remind me that no matter how much progress I feel I've made or how many low-pain days I may have, I am not in control of my own body—not really. I never have been, and I might never be. On the bad pain days, my illnesses and the pain control me. They decide if I leave my house. They decide what I can and cannot eat. And it is these days that paralyze me—both physically and mentally—and leave me questioning why I'm even here at all.

Some people reading this may ask: Why don't you get a roommate? What if someone were there with you? People have been there with me before—there's nothing they can do either. And it somehow makes me feel worse when someone is there and forced to witness it all. As badly as I crave someone being there with me, telling me I can get through it, it also often feels easier to face it alone. People don't always know how to react when something like this happens. And I get it! Hell, I wouldn't either if the roles were reversed. What do you do for someone who is screaming in pain but doesn't want to go to the hospital because she knows they won't do a damn thing for her? Sometimes in the past, when this happened around other people, having them there became more of a burden than a comfort, because suddenly not only was I trying to deal with this pain and talk myself through it, now another person was there asking me to talk them through it as well. And I can't. I can't tell them how to help me or what to do because *there is nothing I can do*.

There is not a single drug available to me on the market that can cause this type of pain to vanish. And believe me, I've tried to find one. I have gone down the pharmaceutical path—prescription-strength ibuprofen and Tramadol. I've done Valium and hormone replacement therapies. But for this type of pain, it's like putting a Band-Aid over a bullet hole. I've tried the holistic approach as well. Sure, I've found some things that help make me more comfortable, but no matter how many needles I have in my body during another acupuncture session, or how many supplements I take every day, the bad days don't disappear. The attacks don't stop happening.

So I can't tell the people around me when a bad day happens how to make the pain stop or how to make it easier for me because there aren't answers to those questions. On the bad days, nothing touches the pain. Nothing comes close. And that realization is scary. So scary, in fact, that if I had to choose whether to face these attacks alone or with someone, I would never choose to face them alone. But inevitably when someone else is there and facing an attack with me, I end up feeling the weight of guilt for days.

It's an interesting concept, that somehow the pain ravaging my body makes *me* feel guilty, as if I'm not the one dealing with it. But it's true—guilt consumes me after a bad flare-up if I have someone with me. Despite knowing for a fact that this pain and these illnesses are not my fault, that's hard to remember on the bad days. I begin to blame myself and then feel ashamed that I caused someone else to pause their life to help me through something that my brain is telling me I *caused*.

I think this because it is the messaging I have always received: that this is somehow my fault. Because these illnesses are so misunderstood and have no cures, most medical professionals I've seen over the years are just guessing what might help. And that guessing comes out as blame. *You should have a stricter diet. You should do more yoga. You should be taking this supplement. You should never eat sugar again. You should sleep more, but in this exact position. If you sleep on your side, you will make it worse. If you use the wrong kind of laundry detergent or shower gel, you will make it worse.* If only I tried a little bit harder, or did a little bit more to help, perhaps I wouldn't be in pain.

The pain and the aftermath of an attack are extremely jarring—not just physically, but emotionally. *I* don't want to experience it. It takes me days, sometimes weeks, to recover from an attack like this. Why would I want to put someone else through that? How could I ask that of anyone?

If there's one thing endometriosis has made me really, really good at, it's considering myself a burden. It doesn't help that in past relationships, I have often felt like one. Sometimes I feel like a bull in a china shop—as if everywhere I go is somehow torn up after I leave. My mere existence feels like a chore: I can't eat or drink certain things; sitting on hard surfaces for too long will cause me to be in pain for days; traveling is hard; drinking alcohol is out of the question, unless I just accept the fact that I will be in more pain than usual the next morning. I am always toeing the line between needing to ask for certain allowances in order to make my life more comfortable and not wanting to say a damn thing, pretending I have no limitations.

I don't want my life to be this way. I don't want to have to ask the waiter to list every single ingredient in a vegetarian patty to make sure it doesn't have something that can cause a flare. I don't want to have to ask the men sleeping in my bed with me if they can please grab me my heating pad or a joint. I don't want any of this. But I never got a choice in the matter. The truth is, I could write an entire book, not just a chapter, dedicated to the impact that endometriosis alone has had on my entire life, and it still wouldn't be enough to cover all the ways in which it has affected me. It's hard not to feel like a burden when the pain you have to live with each and every day is, well, such a goddamn burden.

Of course, it's easier now, on the other side of the attack, to gain perspective and know that despite how awful these occurrences are and how unbearable they have made so many of my days, they are not all my life is. But that they're even a part of it at all is a hard pill to swallow.

* * *

You never forget the first time you lose control over your own body. I didn't know what endometriosis was at the time. I was fourteen years old and home alone. I had just gone on a run outside, trying to get in shape for my upcoming basketball season. While running, I felt a cramp start to form in my abdomen. Within minutes it was so severe that I could no longer stand up straight. I made it into my house and collapsed on the living room floor. When my mom got home from the grocery store, I was dialing 911 on the cordless landline next to me. I didn't know what was happening, but I was sure that it meant I was dying.

It's hard to describe this pain after the fact, which is what makes it so frustrating. You can tell someone that you fantasize about knocking yourself out by throwing your head against the closest dresser, or that you wish for death to take you just so the pain will stop, but unless you witness this type of attack, it's often unimaginable. It's even unimaginable for me most of the time, and I've experienced it countless times now. The body has a way of making us forget things that cause such great pain. It's our body's own defense mechanism—and it's a good one, for the most part. But every time I feel that familiar ache forming in my abdomen, panic rises in my chest as my body starts to remember—and gets really fucking scared.

After the first time I completely lost control of my body due to severe pain, I wrote it off as a freak incident. By the time my mother got home, my pain had started to subside a bit. As my body began to forget the pain, so did I—until it happened again. The second time I lost control of my body was again after running. It once again started out feeling like a relatively normal cramp, albeit more intense. But by the time my feet

stopped hitting the pavement and my knees forced themselves
to the ground while I wrapped my arms around my abdomen
trying to squeeze the pain away, it was a full-blown attack. I
remember crawling into my best friend's house and writhing
around on her living room floor. We were, again, home alone.
By the time her parents got home, I was doing better, but still
in pain. We explained to her mother what had happened.
She said it sounded like I had cramps and gave me Midol. I
thought what I had experienced had been more severe than
menstrual cramps—after all, I literally thought I was going to
die, and by now I had experienced cramping with my period.
None of my cramps had ever felt like that. Plus I wasn't even
on my period. But I was relatively new to having periods and
wasn't sure if I was just misunderstanding how they worked.
Once again, I brushed it off and didn't really think about it
again. That is, until the next time.

This would happen on and off, every couple of months or
so, with no real rhyme or reason, until I eventually ended up
at urgent care at age fifteen. I was told that I was just an emotional teenager. A few years later, I ended up in the emergency
room where I was told that I should take Advil. Yes, Advil. The
over-the-counter drug. As if Advil were the cure for the attacks that kept happening in my body. As if it were ever that
simple. As if I had never considered doing anything about the
pain at all. I mostly stopped asking for help from doctors until
years later, when I was no longer able to function and had no
options left.

It's hard to believe that a disease that is so unnervingly
common can cause this amount of pain for people, sometimes
on a daily basis, and yet the best option we have, according to
doctors, is either completely stopping our hormones or putting our bodies through an invasive surgery—one that is rarely

covered in full by insurance, requires weeks of recovery time, and is by no means a cure. Endometriosis is not rare. It is also not just a bad period. It is not just some abdominal swelling or trouble digesting. It is not just deep-in-your-bones exhaustion, or horrifically painful sex. It is all this and *more*. It is debilitating. It is the most physically painful thing I have ever experienced, and it is also the most mentally painful thing I've ever had to deal with. It hurts. It hurts so bad. And every time it hurts, I am reminded that there is next to nothing I can do about it. I am reminded that there is no cure. I feel as if I am shackled to this pain. Even on my relatively good days, I am chained down by the fear of when the pain will return. I am like a hamster on a wheel from which I cannot figure a way off. Round and round I go—having a horrible pain day, coming out of it, trying to move on, then having another horrible pain day and starting the cycle all over again.

And despite desperately begging and pleading for help from the medical community on and off for years, here I am at age twenty-eight, still figuring it out on my own. I am not only dealing with the burden of the pain on a daily basis, but I am also solely responsible for figuring out how to make my life livable despite it! We all are. We are not given the help we so desperately need—and deserve—from doctors or medical professionals of any kind, so we must shoulder the burden of being our own caregivers as well. It is exhausting. It is overwhelming.

And it is incessant. I barely passed biology in high school but suddenly I was tasked, as a teenager, with figuring out how to fight back against a disease I knew next to nothing about. I have spent hours creating food diary after food diary to pinpoint my triggers and connect the dots of the symptoms I was experiencing. I have watched countless YouTube videos on pelvic floor stretches I could do to help ease the pain in my lower back. I have done my best to read (and comprehend!) medical study after medical study on the effects that certain supplements or prescription drugs could or could not have on my illnesses. I have read every blog post I could find about vaginal steaming to help reduce severe period pain, and more than two hundred comments from people around the world describing their experience with drinking celery juice every morning. I have pored over reviews of different dilator sets, and bought three different books about how to "cure pelvic pain once and for all." Every time I felt I had figured something out or made progress with one pain, another would appear, and I would be back on that hamster wheel, spinning faster and faster, until I felt like I could no longer breathe. And each time my new approach to treating and managing my symptoms would fail, I would have no one to blame but myself.

No, these illnesses are not my fault. But when you're the only person doing anything to combat them, and you have a medical community that downplays the severity of your symptoms and writes them off as "no big deal," you start to feel like you have no one else to blame.

No matter how many times I tell people that endometriosis affects me, in no small part, every single day of my life, I still feel like people don't understand. And I acknowledge that it is hard to imagine for a variety of different reasons. I don't blame anyone. I can hardly wrap my mind around it most of the time, and I'm living with it. But it is absolutely vital that people understand the deep burden of living with this condition. So I've outlined an average week in my life to help people get a better sense of what my day to day is like. Before we even dive into this, it's crucial for me to remind you that I am one of the very, very lucky ones who not only has health insurance, but access to cannabis and a disposable income that allows for treatments such as acupuncture and physical therapy. And yet, despite all that, I am still in some form of pain every single day of my life.

A typical week in my life with endometriosis:

Monday:

5:37 A.M.: An ache in my lower back wakes me up before my alarm. I can't remember the last time I actually slept through a night without waking up due to some discomfort in my body. I crawl out of bed and go to the bathroom to pee because I know that if I do not, my bladder will continue keeping me up with a dull ache.

6:30 A.M.: Because I am up so early and actually able to walk without being hunched over in pain today, I decide to take my dog on a hike. The trail I usually do is a two-mile loop and takes me around forty minutes. Hiking isn't the best thing for my body—I have a lot of stress on my pelvic floor muscles as it is, and hiking can cause that to intensify. But because hiking is one of the few physical activities I can do these days, I like to go. Plus, being outside in nature with my dog almost makes me feel normal. Almost. I go on the hike and then head to work.

2:00 P.M.: I still have three hours of work to get through, but my lower back is screaming in pain. My pain is worse today because I neglected to do my stretches. I don't have the luxury of getting a break on things like this. I rarely feel like doing stretches after getting home from a hike, but I always pay for that later.

5:00 P.M.: When the end of the workday rolls around, I collapse into my car and almost cry from the relief of knowing that I will soon be home on my couch, able to smoke weed and do my best to forget the pain raging inside my body.

5:45 P.M.: By the time I get home and take my dog outside for the shortest walk of her life, I can hardly stand up straight. I smoke as much weed as my body will allow. Cannabis is currently the only thing I rely on for pain relief. While it does significantly help me on bad pain days, it's certainly not a cure, and it's hardly a solution. As much fun as it can be to be stoned out of my gourd watching *90 Day Fiancé* on my couch with my dog, having to get stoned out of your mind multiple times a week in order to stand being in your own body is not something I would wish on anyone.

6:15 P.M.: It's not even 7 P.M. yet, but I know I'm not leaving my couch for the rest of the night. As I drift into a semi-comatose state from the weed and the pain, I try not to think about how I am being forced to spend yet another evening on my couch with an abdomen that feels as if it is being ripped apart from the inside out.

Tuesday:

5:30 A.M.: After spending hours on my couch in a pain haze the night before, I am anxious to get out of my apartment, and I wake up before my alarm. The pain is still lingering, but it's much less severe than it was the night before, and I am grateful.

For the most part, my pain is at its least severe in the mornings and then gains momentum as the day goes on. But I don't think about that this morning. All I think about is the fact that it's tapered off for now.

7:03 A.M.: I take my dog on a long walk through the neighborhood. This time, as soon as I get back inside, I do my stretches. I am exhausted, but since I can rarely drink caffeine without it increasing my pain levels, I decide to get a smoothie on my way to work instead. One of the biggest symptoms of my endometriosis is trouble eating because I am almost constantly nauseous, and because I constantly feel bloated and swollen. I rely heavily on cannabis— namely CBD capsules—in order to have an appetite to eat every day. Without cannabis, I would rarely be able to eat, and even if I did, I certainly wouldn't enjoy food as much. But sometimes, even when cannabis gives me an appetite, as soon as I eat, my stomach swells.

8:30 A.M.: After getting a smoothie and making sure it has ginger in it so that it doesn't irritate my stomach further, I head to acupuncture. If I could, I would go to acupuncture twice a week. It is one of the few things that helps my pain levels and reduces inflammation in my body. But, even with insurance coverage, I still have to pay thirty dollars out of pocket every time I go. And while I can afford that for the most part, it adds up, as does the time it takes to go for an hour appointment twice a week. I spend an hour and a half with my acupuncturist today, an extra thirty minutes while she does her best to ease the swelling that I feel in every inch of my body. I fall asleep, and when I wake up, I feel more at ease.

10:05 A.M.: I go straight to work after acupuncture, and even though I'm feeling physically better today, I feel mentally exhausted from being in so much pain the day before. I somehow make it through the day and sit through meetings, contributing when I can.

4:46 P.M.: I go straight home after work and take my dog on a walk before lying on my couch and—once again—getting high in order to make myself feel more comfortable. I watch 90 *Day Fiancé* until I fall asleep.

Wednesday:

7:00 A.M.: The week is barely halfway through and I'm already questioning how I can make it until Friday, and how I've ever managed to work a full forty-hour week in my life. My body feels heavy. The pain is just enough today that I notice it with every step I take, but not enough for me to feel like I have a reason to stay home in bed. I am extremely—I cannot emphasize this enough—lucky to have a career that does not require me to be in an office every day. But despite this, I don't feel any less guilty anytime I have to stay home because of a pain flare, and I try to avoid it. It's a constant game I play with myself—stay home today and hope it doesn't get worse by tomorrow? Or push through in case it *is* worse tomorrow?

9:13 A.M.: By the time I make it to work, it's as if I can feel the inflammation in every inch of my body. It's a difficult sensation to describe, like little red fire ants eating you all over. On days like this, I constantly have the urge to unzip my skin. The best I can do is try to make myself comfortable and get through the day's tasks so that I can get home sooner and take a cannabis bath.

11:03 A.M.: I take four 25-milligram CBD capsules and go into the office bathroom to rub CBD balm on my abdomen and lower back. I try to limit the amount of human interaction I have because I can feel myself growing angrier by the second. It's not anyone's fault that I am in pain. And it's not anyone's fault that they are not in pain. But knowing that doesn't stop me from becoming angry sometimes. It can feel so unfair to watch as other people seemingly glide through life with so few limitations. It can feel like a personal attack to hear the person in front of you at the water fountain talking about how hungover they are, or watch as your coworkers all pitch in and order something you would never be able to eat for lunch. The anger is not reasonable. It's not rational. But neither is being in pain every single day.

4:30 P.M.: I somehow make it through most of the day, only crying in the bathroom once, and get in my car to leave. Tonight, instead of just going home to my couch to sit, I head to therapy. Again, I am one of the fortunate ones: Not only am I able to see a therapist on a regular basis, but I also have one I've been working with for more than three years now. My therapist has an autoimmune disorder, and though it's not the same as having Vagina Problems, there's a level of understanding there that simply cannot be replaced.

6:00 P.M.: Therapy can often feel repetitive to me. It's rare that I can get through a therapy session without bringing up how unfair it feels to have to live this life—a life of pain. For the most part, I stopped a long time ago trying to find a reason why I'm living it and instead just try to focus on staying in the present and taking one day at a time. On this particular day in therapy, I talk to my therapist about the awful pain flare I had a couple of nights prior. I tell her how draining it is to feel constantly as if I am being forced to miss out on life.

She says we should reframe how I think about this. She says that realistically I *could* have gotten off my couch. Would it have been difficult? Yes. A bad idea? Absolutely. But she continues, suggesting I try not to think of it as the pain "winning" or me "losing" another day of my life. She suggests that I think of it as a choice—like I am surrendering. It gives me some of the power back. Sure, I could have gotten off the couch, but because that's not what my body needed, I made the decision not to. My pain didn't win—I surrendered. I took note of the situation, listened to my body, and did what was best for it. And that's fucking empowering.

8:17 P.M.: Since this conversation with my therapist, I've done my best to remember this empowering reframing every time I feel as if I'm being forced—yet again—to miss out on life because of pain out of my control. I'm not losing. I'm giving in. My pain does not control me. I control how I react to my pain. I take a hot cannabis bath and go to bed. I only wake up once that night.

Thursday:

7:33 A.M.: I wake up feeling a bit lighter after therapy the night before and remind myself that it is almost the weekend. I have acupuncture again this morning. I usually only go once a week, but my pain has been so bad lately. I feel a twinge of guilt when I remember that I will have to show up to work a bit late yet again, but I try to squash that thought as soon as it enters my mind. I say the same things over and over to myself, almost like a mantra. *I didn't ask for this. I'm doing the best I can. Anyone else in my position would do the same. Honestly, they might not even show up to work at all.* I don't know if that's true or not, but I tell myself it is anyway.

8:26 A.M.: I get my morning smoothie—I rarely eat anything else for breakfast because of nausea—and go to acupuncture. My acupuncturist asks me how I'm feeling today—but she knows how I am going to respond. It's always the same: *Not good.* Anyone who tells you that acupuncture doesn't hurt is lying. When you find a good acupuncturist who knows what they are doing and knows exactly what spots to hit on your body, you will absolutely feel the needle enter your skin. But it's not a stabbing sensation—it's nothing like a shot. It's a pressure point being hit. That's how you know it's working. I like going to acupuncture and feeling that pain. It distracts me from the other pain, and also reminds me that my pain is real and not the figment of my imagination my brain sometimes still tries to convince me it is. I spend an hour and a half with my acupuncturist and leave with less aching in my lower back.

5:23 P.M.: I make it through my workday with little issue, and when I get home from work, I find myself with the energy to take Pepper on an evening stroll to get dinner somewhere. Tomorrow is Friday, I tell myself, and the week is almost done. Despite feeling like I wouldn't be able to do it, I've nearly done it yet again—worked a full week without missing a day. I get a vegan jackfruit burrito bowl and take a cannabis edible to give myself the appetite to eat it. I fall asleep soon after, resting easier knowing that the weekend is close.

Friday:

8:09 A.M.: Although it is Friday and arguably the easiest workday of the week, I have a hard time getting out of bed. I'm exhausted, both mentally and physically. Spending thirty minutes on Instagram as soon as I woke up this morning didn't help. It likely wouldn't help anyone have a good day, but it especially didn't help me when I saw story after story and picture after picture of people living life without endometriosis pain. I don't get out of bed until after 8 A.M., although I need to be at work by 9. I won't have time to stop for a morning smoothie, which is stupid on my part because then I'll no doubt end up trying to eat some sort of free breakfast at work, which will likely contain gluten or sugar—both of which make my inflammation worse. I don't feel like I have the energy to both take a shower and ingest my daily dose of vitamins and supplements, so I choose the vitamin route and decide that I don't care how oily my hair looks.

8:47 A.M.: My abdomen feels swollen even though I haven't put anything in it besides half a vegan burrito bowl in the last twelve hours. I opt for stretchy yoga pants for the third time this week because the thought of anything else touching my abdomen makes me want to cry. *It's just eight hours, then you can lie around as much as you want.* I am going to be late to work. I wish I had the energy to care.

9:17 A.M.: I make it to work and go through the motions. Everything feels like a blur. I do my best to keep the clouds in my head at bay and stay focused.

2:07 P.M.: I feel so spent that I can't imagine continuing to sit up straight or even lifting my head.

5:16 P.M.: By the time I make it home from work, I am so tired that I choose to do nothing but sit on my couch and get high—both because I am in pain and because I am deeply sad about being in pain. Despite all the coping mechanisms I've learned over the years, none of them seems to be working. So I give in to the sadness and hopelessness and just let myself cry. Pepper licks my tears.

8:03 P.M.: I go to bed after taking CBD plus melatonin supplements and tell myself that tomorrow is a new day.

Saturday:

7:23 A.M.: I made plans with a friend to hike today but as soon as I wake up, I know I won't be able to. I have such bad bladder pain, it feels as if I drank acid before going to sleep the night before. I spend a few minutes trying to figure out what I did to cause this pain. I never come up with an answer. As the pain becomes more and more obvious the more my body awakens, I start panicking and go down a list of things I need to do immediately. Step 1: Get food. I know I will be in no mental or physical state to acquire food later, and because I had no energy during the week to grocery shop, I have next to nothing edible in my apartment. Sometimes I order groceries or rely on food delivery services, but this requires the energy to get up off the couch to get the food, as my apartment building's buzzer is broken. And since none of the delivery services are open right now anyway, I drag myself out of bed and feel the stabbing in my abdomen with every step I take.

7:47 A.M.: I take Pepper out for a quick pee and scold her for taking too long. I immediately feel bad when I see her innocent eyes look up at me, confused about why she isn't being given more time to sniff the grass this morning. I wish I could explain to her how much I hurt. I wish I could make her understand that if I could change my life and be a dog owner without pain who could take her on endless walks whenever she wanted, I would do it in a second. I can feel tears start to form in my eyes and know that I have to hurry because I am close to my breaking point.

8:01 A.M.: I get in my car and go to the closest grocery store, where I grab whatever food I can find that is least likely to hurt me but is also easy to consume. On days like today, I don't have the energy to cook. Heating something up in the microwave is almost too much. I spend a total of twelve minutes in the grocery store. It feels like two hours. I am one of five customers at such an early hour on a Saturday.

8:13 A.M.: I rush home, and as soon as I walk through the door, I get completely naked and put on my biggest and comfiest robe. I can't stand to have any clothing clinging to my lower back or abdomen today. I put my rice-filled heating pad in the microwave and start applying cannabis rub all over my body. I stick a cannabis suppository up my vagina. I grab a joint; take an edible; get my TENS unit, which is a little handheld device that sends small electrical currents to targeted body parts, relieving some of my pain; some snacks; and lots of water, and put it all on the table next to me on the couch. My heating pad needs at least five minutes in the microwave to heat up, and it feels like the longest five minutes of my life.

8:20 A.M.: By the time the heating pad is ready and I am on the couch smoking and applying heat to my abdomen, I can barely lift my head. I know that I will not be able to move from the couch for the rest of the day. It is barely 8:30 A.M. and my day is over before it began. I know I should text a friend and ask for help. I know I should try to put something on Netflix to distract myself. I know I should do anything to try to keep myself from falling into the state of depression that so often accompanies this type of pain. But I can't. I won't. I don't do anything. I just sit on my couch smoking as much weed as I can handle until I barely remember my own name. And even then, I can still feel the ache in my back.

4:00 P.M.: I stay like that, on the couch staring off into space, for the next eight hours. I eventually somehow manage to take Pepper out for a short walk. When I'm in the elevator on the way back up to my apartment, I see myself in the mirror. I look as awful as I feel. I can see my swollen stomach. I look pregnant. It feels worse than it looks, but the fact that it's visible somehow makes me feel worse. I start to cry but try hard not to let the tears drop from my eyes. I feel fragile—like a piece of delicate antique glassware that is seconds away from breaking. I fear that if I let a single tear fall or acknowledge my emotions at all, I will shatter completely and will never be able to piece myself back together again. I try to repeat my mantras back to myself. *You are surrendering. Your pain does not own you. This will not last forever. You will get through this, you always do.* But none of it works. I don't even believe them anymore.

4:15 P.M.: I use all my willpower to text my therapist and ask if she can see me tomorrow on short notice. I turn on the TV and try to find something to watch that will make my brain stop fucking thinking. Nothing works. I try to read a book but after rereading the same sentence twelve times in a row, I give up.

7:00 P.M.: I am spiraling deeper and deeper into this dangerous pattern of thought. *This is all your life is, just a series of bad pain days over and over and over again. What is the point? How will you be able to do this for another ten years? Why would anyone ever want to spend their life with you if this is how it is? How would you ever be able to start a family if you wanted one? What is the point of your life? Why do you even exist if you're just going to be in pain all the time? People are tired of hearing you complain about it. It's endless. It's all you talk about. It's all you are.* I try so hard to tell the thoughts to stop. I try so hard to get them to shut up. But I can't. I don't know how anymore. Any strength or fight I had in me earlier this week is gone. All I feel now is pain . . . and sadness. I once again feel tears forming in my eyes. This time, I don't have the energy to try to stop them. As they begin to spill out heavier and heavier, I start to unravel. Before long, I'm sobbing, and Pepper is trying to lick the tears from my face. I wonder if my neighbors can hear me, if they think I'm crazy or need professional help.

8:03 P.M.: An hour passes and I finally feel as if I have no tears left to cry. My phone buzzes. It's my therapist. *I'll see you at 11 A.M. tomorrow, Lara. Please be kind to yourself until then.* After letting myself break down, I feel numb. I eventually fall asleep on my couch cradling my heating pad, with Pepper pressed up against my stomach.

Sunday:

7:03 A.M.: I wake up early, feeling raw and sore from sleeping on the couch. Pepper is still pressed into my stomach, curled up into a little ball. Seeing her makes me cry all over again, but this time it's a different sort of cry. I thank her for being with me during the bad days.

7:30 A.M.: I'm feeling better today, so I take Pepper on a long walk and let her sniff extra grass this morning to make up for yesterday. Although I feel physically better today, I still feel extremely raw after yesterday. Being sick and having an illness like endometriosis is so much more than just dealing with physical pain. The emotional pain feels more difficult to deal with most of the time.

11:00 A.M.: I go see my therapist and cry to her for an hour straight about how I feel as if I can no longer do this. When I leave, I feel a little bit lighter, but also exhausted.

12:00 P.M.: Back home, I take a four-hour nap with Pep by my side.

4:00 P.M.: When I wake up, it is practically evening and my weekend is almost over. I can never decide which I prefer—for my bad pain days to be on the weekend so I don't have to feel guilty about missing work, or for the bad pain days to happen during the week so I don't have to sacrifice my weekends.

6:45 P.M.: I try to process my feelings about the weekend but instead end up watching another episode of 90 Day Fiancé and sexting men from dating apps. It's nice sometimes to sext and pretend that I am not a person who is stuck on her couch for the thirty-ninth hour in a row due to pain out of her control. When I sext I can be whoever I want. And I always choose to be someone who is not in pain.

* * *

Despite all I have done and continue to do to fight back against the pain in my body, I never feel like I'm doing enough. I could spend hours a week attending physical therapy and acupuncture, eating clean, stretching my limbs, taking my vitamins and supplements, and getting enough sleep, and still wake up in pain. It never feels like enough, because it never actually is. I often wonder if it ever will be. There are so many layers to endometriosis. It's the physical pain, the mental pain, the deep-in-your-bones feeling of hopelessness, and the fight it instills in you that doesn't allow you to give up, even on the worst days, when you feel like you have nothing else to give. It's a pain unlike anything I've ever known before—and one that, no matter how hard I try to forget it, always haunts me.

Most of the time these days I think of my life in two parts: the Lara before endometriosis, and the Lara after endometriosis entered my life. Try as I might not to let this disease define me, I don't get much choice in the matter. It's hard to ignore something or pretend it isn't happening when it is always there, reminding you. I am a lot of things, and I do a lot of things in my life—but I am not exaggerating when I tell you that it is almost impossible to think of a time in the last decade of my life that endometriosis has not impacted in some way. That's not to say that all my life consists of is endometriosis pain or thinking about endometriosis. I'd like to believe that I live a pretty full life regardless. But no matter how hard I try, it's still there, even on the good days. I hardly remember the Lara before endometriosis. I genuinely can't remember what it's like to not feel the familiar ache in my abdomen, or the searing pain in my bladder after taking a sip of alcohol.

In the past people have asked me: If you were given the choice, would you get rid of the pain? I always thought this was an asinine question to ask. Like . . . yes. Are you fucking kidding me? Of course I would choose to get rid of the pain in my body. But on my good days, I sometimes ponder this question a bit more and wonder. Despite the havoc endometriosis has wreaked on my life, it's also shown me my own strength. It has forced me to face my biggest fears time and time again and prove to myself that I can get through them. It has given me the beautiful ability to experience not only sympathy for others who are suffering, but true empathy. It has made me a fighter—not just against this disease, but against any and all bullshit in my life. It has forced me to appreciate the little moments in life a bit more, because to me, they really are so fleeting. It has forced me to appreciate my resilience, even when I am not feeling particularly durable. And because of endometriosis, I know how to listen to my body. Despite all this, if given the choice, I would obviously still choose not to deal with it. I would always choose that. Always. But in many ways, I would not be who I am today if I did not have endometriosis. And although it's difficult to see on my bad days—the person I am is pretty fucking great.

4

What It's Like to Live in Constant Pain

Chronic pain is a difficult concept to understand, even for those of us living with it. The idea of something that constantly recurs is hard to grapple with. But it's especially hard to grasp when the thing is pain. Most of what we're taught about health is that you're either dying or just haven't found the right medication to take yet. There hasn't been much room left for what's in between, the place where those of us with chronic pain or chronic illnesses are forced to exist. Because even if we manage to receive a reason for our pain, the reason doesn't come with a solution. So we remain in between—obsessed with the idea that a solution to our pain is somewhere out there while also doing our best to accept that we've done everything we can.

I'll never forget the moment I realized my illnesses weren't going to go away. The moment that, no matter how hard I tried, I couldn't deny it anymore—that my illnesses and the pain that came with them weren't just going to fade away into the abyss like I had hoped over and over again on my worst pain days. They were here to stay despite everything I'd done to make them go away.

I had just gone through yet another failed attempt at finding a treatment to put an end to my chronic pain once and for all. This time it was a combination of herbs, acupuncture, deep-tissue laser treatments, and chiropractic work. I had already gone the surgery route. I had tried prescriptions. I'd had energy work done. I'd changed my diet approximately twenty thousand times. I felt like I had done it all. Everything I could get my hands on—that didn't come with myriad side effects, at least. This time I had been feeling some improvement. I hadn't completely lost consciousness during my period for a few months, and I had a few days with more energy throughout the month. But then, all at once, my pain came rushing back like water overflowing a broken dam after a storm. The treatments hadn't worked. None of them. Some had helped for a little bit, some even gave me lasting relief in one way or another. But at the end of the day, I was still sick and still having bad pain days. And it finally dawned on me that there might be absolutely nothing I could do about that. I had once again run out of options. And I was once again back on my couch, in so much pain that getting up wasn't possible. That's when it all hit me.

Of course I had known, deep down, long before this day, that these illnesses weren't a fluke or some sort of test that I would either pass or fail. But on this particular day, whatever gates I had managed to put in place between myself and the realization that I had chronic, incurable illnesses came crashing down. Suddenly I felt like I was being swept away in a wild river current. I tried desperately to cling to the things that usually gave me comfort as if they were a tree branch or a root on the side of the river, but no matter how many times I told myself that medicine was constantly changing or that the world was full of knowledge and information that I maybe just didn't have access to yet . . . I couldn't stop the spiral. It felt like I had placed all my eggs in this basket, the basket that was supposed to fucking fix me, and the eggs were shattered right before my eyes.

Although I certainly had days prior to this one where I was upset and feeling adrift about living with these illnesses, I'd always done my best to avoid giving those thoughts too much space in my mind. I've been afraid of letting myself really *go there*. And by *there*, I mean the place where I acknowledge how I actually feel about living with illnesses that currently have no cure. Because really, it's not just about finding a way to continue on with my illnesses and the constant swelling in my abdomen and the ache in my back. It's also trying to find a way to live my life in spite of it all.

I've always feared that if I admit what's really going on and acknowledge that these illnesses actually do impact my life in some way every single day, and that there is currently no cure or magic pill that I can take to make that pain go away, maybe I'll never actually come back from it. Because it's not just admitting that they affect my life every day. It's also admitting how I *feel* about that. And admitting that would mean admitting that sometimes, more often than not, I genuinely despise my life. I despise that I was forced to live with such pain and never given a real reason why. I despise that there are other people on this earth who do not have to live with this pain. I despise the way it makes me feel—both physically and emotionally. I despise the way it is *always* there, lingering, no matter how hard I try, or how strictly I keep my diet, or how good I think I feel. I loathe the fact that this pain has infiltrated the most intimate moments of my life and caused me such agony that sometimes a part of me doesn't even want to try anymore, at all . . . ever.

I can barely stand to think of the moments in my life that have been overshadowed by this pain. And I certainly can't stand to think of the many more moments it will likely ruin in my future, when I am forced to remind myself, again, that there is no cure *and that nothing I have done so far truly makes this shit go away.* In fact, my pain has only gotten worse with age. Sure, I'm more accustomed to it now. I know what CBD balms to use, and I know when a pain flare is here to stay for a while. But no number of years spent with this pain will ever get me to a place where I am okay with what it does to me. I still feel the fear in my chest at the thought of going through another attack. I still find myself wondering if this one will be the one that happens while I am driving to work, or when I am walking through the airport. I wonder if this will be the one that causes me to fall and hit my head, rendering me even more useless than I already feel. Admitting these things means admitting that sometimes, more often than not these days, I don't want to live this life anymore. I don't want it to be this way. But I know I've been given no choice.

I'm not really in denial. I've read the medical studies. I've seen the statistics. I've watched as doctor after doctor does their best to come up with a solution to my myriad problems. I've gone to all the appointments, and I've seen the charts meant for marking my improvements stay the same month after month, year after year. I've read the stories of other people with my illnesses. And I've felt my own pain inside my body too many times not to have an inkling of what's going on. I know that in many ways, the odds of somehow suddenly being free of these illnesses and my pain altogether are bleak. The pain is too widespread, too deep in my nerves, and too ingrained in my body at this point to just disappear one day. My body is used to it by now. It only knows pain. If the endometriosis were to suddenly disappear one day, I wouldn't just stop being in pain. My muscles wouldn't just bounce back and begin working properly. But knowing this and allowing these thoughts to infiltrate my mind and take up space are two different things.

In the past, these realizations have come and gone. On the day I'm speaking of, however, the dam broke, and suddenly I didn't know how to swim anymore. No matter how hard I tried to remind myself that medical advancements happen all the time, or that I was going to get through this flare and feel okay again, I was no longer sure how to keep my head above water, and I was starting to question whether it was worthwhile to keep trying.

* * *

Living with chronic pain feels like you're in a constant battle. You are never able to put down your weapons and just relax. You have to be persistently on alert. Every decision I make is somehow impacted by my illnesses. Even when I tell myself that they do not define me, they find a way to remind me that actually, sometimes they do. I can't get dressed in the morning without taking my illnesses into account. Hell, I can't even wake up in the morning without immediately feeling an ache in my lower back—and that's if I've slept through the night without being woken by discomfort. Even if I try my best to ignore the pain, it follows me. If I wear the wrong type of underwear, it could mean that I'll be in so much pain by 3 P.M. that I'll have to leave work early and miss my afternoon meetings. Thongs can burn in hell. Boy shorts were created by the devil.

And trendy tight-fitting, high-waisted jeans were invented just to ruin my life, I think.

It's not just the little things each day that start to wear me down, though. When deciding how to celebrate my birthday, I first have to check my period tracking app to see what day of my cycle my birthday lands on and plan accordingly, based on what my pain levels might be. I can't go to brunch without having to dissect every menu item to find something that will cause me the least amount of discomfort and won't require me to leave the gathering early to go lie on my couch and get stoned because I'm in so much pain from drinking a fucking mimosa. Going on a hike and not doing my stretches afterward? Pain. Drinking caffeine? Pain. Eating a food that sounds good but somehow contains a trigger that I didn't even fucking know about? Pain. Pain. Pain. It's always there, even when I do my best to keep it away.

While most of my feelings regarding the chronic pain I have lived with for more than a decade now can be best described as "fucking sad," I'm also angry. And that's something I don't think I talk about enough—the anger that accompanies a life of pain. There are thousands of emotions that I have felt in regard to my chronic pain. Some of them I don't even have a name for. But anger is one of the most persistent. It's also the one that makes me feel the most ashamed. The truth is, as sad as I am to feel as if I have no control over my life because I live with chronic pain, that sadness sometimes feels small compared to how angry I can be. I want to shatter my phone when I see people posting running-app screenshots of the miles they've run. I want to fucking scream sometimes when I hear someone complain about having to take Advil for their period cramps. I've had to fight the urge to pour the rest of the water in my glass on coworkers who complain about how hungover they are on a Monday morning and how they should be given the day off. I occasionally feel myself start to shake when I overhear a conversation among friends about how hard dating is for them. It's not fair. I know that. It's not rational. But then again, neither is being in constant pain.

Sometimes when I feel that familiar swelling starting up in my abdomen, I have the urge to rip my insides out. I fantasize about peeling apart my skin and removing every part of me that hurts. I wonder what it would be like to open up my own body with a knife and look at the organs inside of me that cause me such agony. I wonder what it might be like to look my uterus in the face, or what it would be like to peel the endometriosis away from my intestines. I don't want to just remove it, though. I want to destroy it. I daydream about throwing the endometrium tissue on the ground and pouring gasoline on top of it to watch it burn. I yearn to destroy the illnesses in my body the way I feel they have destroyed me.

When I have these thoughts, they are rooted in deep anger. Anger that has no place to go. I want to yell at someone. I want to tell all my friends to just leave me alone and never speak to me again. I don't want to speak to anyone, not even my closest friends, while simultaneously feeling like I want every single person in my life to come hold me and tell me everything is going to be all right.

When I get angry like this, when I lose that control and the cork pops off, I feel myself start to unravel. I start to feel like I can't do it anymore. I don't know how I can keep doing this. I want a reason for this! I want a reason for this pain. I want someone to be angry at. I want someone, or something, to throw all this emotion at so that I don't have to feel it anymore.

Deep down, I know that I am not really mad at my friends.

I'm not really mad at the person I went to one semester of college with for being at a bowling alley drinking a beer on a Saturday night. I'm not really mad at people for complaining about their period cramps, or their hangover, or the trials and tribulations of dating. People are allowed to feel things. People are allowed to be human, to be who they are. I know that. I also know that really, deep down, I'm mad at these diseases. But no matter how angry I am at them, no matter how much I tell them to go away or to leave me alone . . . they never do. So I get fucking angry again. I'm so angry that sometimes I feel as if I can no longer breathe. I want to scream at these diseases and tell them to go away. I beg them to go away. I try to put up a fight. I throw anger at them and try to show them who is boss. But I don't win. I never win.

I'm tired of feeling it. It never goes away. It never stops. It is constant. It is always in my brain, like a fucking worm, reminding me that I have to live a life that is shrouded with pain for no goddamn reason. Reminding me that I cannot walk up a set of stairs without hurting my body in some way. I cannot do ANYTHING. And the reminders make me panic. They make me feel like lighting a match and watching things burn—which is what my body sometimes feels like. It feels like I slowly crumble into a pile of ash when pain makes my body fall apart again. I want to be mad at my friends for being out at a bar right now. I want to be mad at everyone except my own body because it once again failed me. I can't even make my own decision about how I spend my time.

Try as I might not to define my life by my illnesses and the pain associated with them, it's a constant uphill battle. On one hand, I am very aware that I am a person, not a chronic illness. There are many facets to my life that do not include the pain in my vagina and surrounding areas. But on the other hand, it's a pretty fucking big part of my life. I mean, I feel it *every day.* If you were to have a headache every single day, don't you imagine that you would speak about it? You might wake up and think, "Fuck, I have this damn headache again! That's pretty annoying." When someone asked you how your week was going, you might want to say, "Well, I've had this goddamn headache for DAYS now. It simply won't go away no matter what I do, or how many Advil I take." You might even want to talk about it on social media. And why wouldn't you? It's becoming a large part of your days. It's affecting how you live your life and the activities that you are able to participate in. Of course you want to talk about it!

That's how I feel about my pain. Which is why I do talk about it—both online and in real life. But what I've learned by talking about my experience with chronic pain is that people don't understand that when I talk about it, I am not looking for answers or a solution. Oftentimes I'm not looking for anything. I'm just talking openly about something that is happening in my life. I don't want to live in this anger forever, or even for longer than a day. But I can't pretend it isn't there. I've tried that, believe me. And I only end up feeling angrier in the long run. It feels, to me, as if it's a natural part of the grieving process.

And in many ways, people who live with chronic pain *are* grieving. We are grieving for the lives we could've had, but don't, because of pain. But in the past, when I've shared my frustration or anger or sadness about living with this pain, I've often been met with a lack of understanding. People say things to me, usually the same things over and over again: *Stay positive. It could be worse. At least you don't have *insert random other awful disease here.** I've always been confused by this reaction. I mean, I guess I understand it. People are doing what they think is helpful by reminding me that although I am upset, it could always be worse. It's that sentiment of counting your blessings and choosing to look at the glass as half full. But I think it's bullshit. Telling me that someone somewhere else on earth has a problem that is worse than mine doesn't make me feel better. It certainly doesn't make my vagina hurt any less, or my abdomen feel any less swollen. Really, all it does is succeed in making me feel guilty for the very understandable anger I have about being in pain. I *know* it could be worse. But knowing that other people suffer doesn't make me suffer any less.

* * *

It took me a long time to get to the place where I could talk openly and honestly about my pain, and the way it makes me feel, without feeling as if I'm doing something wrong. I *know* there are worse things in life than dealing with what I am dealing with. I understand that life is full of shit. But what I don't understand is how being reminded of that is supposed to make me feel better. I do not believe that someone's honesty about their pain or heartache is wrong simply because someone else in the world also has heartache. It's not a fucking competition.

The world is shit most of the time, but it's made shittier when we try to talk about our shit and are told that we're not allowed to think of our lives as shit because someone else's shit smells worse. **Shit is shit**. There's a lot of shit—it's a big world, and there's unfortunately room for all our shit. I don't need you or anyone else to try to fix my shit or make it disappear. I don't need you to minimize the very real emotions I am experiencing. I just want the space to talk about it and know that it is okay. I want to say how fucking angry I am that I have never once been able to orgasm without some inkling of pain, immediately afterward or hours later, when my vulva burns with every step I take as it rubs against my underwear. And I don't want that to be diminished or ignored or shamed simply because there are other issues in the world. I just want people to be able to sit with me in that pain. I don't expect them to know what it feels like or to say they understand. I wouldn't ask that of people. All I ask is for the space to feel how I feel. We all deserve that. All of us.

More times than I can count I've been met with disbelief, as if I'm lying about the way my body feels in order to garner sympathy. But even when people *do* believe that I'm not lying about the amount of pain I'm in, they seem to have a hard time believing that I'm doing everything I can to keep the pain at bay.

If it isn't people reminding me that my pain could be worse, so I should just suck it up and stop being a sad, angry girl; or minimizing my pain and telling me it's "making me stronger"; it's people thinking they can fix me. My god. There are always these people. Always. If I had to define what living with a chronic illness is really like, I think it would be this: You are just trying to live your life and do the best you can, but you are constantly bombarded with people who truly believe they know what is best for your body. They, the people who are not living in your body, think they understand it better than you . . . THE PERSON IN THE BODY. And even though you never asked them for help or communicated that you would like advice, they give it to you anyway. And 99.9 percent of the time, it's useless. Not only is it useless, though. It's also downright insulting.

I feel very confident saying that there is not a single person on this planet who is living with a chronic illness who has not attempted to make it better in some way. None of us are just sitting around on our asses day after day hoping that one day the pain will magically disappear. We are trying. When people suggest a million things that we should do to feel better, it can make us feel as if they think we haven't tried at all. *Have you tried yoga? Have you tried standing on your head seventeen times a day? Have you tried taking the very common and popular over-the-counter medicine referred to as "Advil"? Have you tried breathing? Have you considered seeing a DoCtOr? Maybe try drinking some celery juice?? Maybe just, I don't know, stop being sad? LOL! Have you considered going into the forest and lying under a tree and letting the sunlight hit you three to seven times a day while rubbing dirt on your arms?*

Have *you* tried shutting the fuck up????????

I've spent too many hours, days, and months wondering why some people have such strong reactions when it comes to someone, like myself, speaking openly about their chronic pain and the emotions surrounding it. Over the years I've concluded that some of the responses I receive that imply I'm not doing enough, or I'm just not eating or drinking the right things, are rooted in fear. The idea that there are human beings on this earth who are living with persistent pain and discomfort with no cure and little solution is scary to those who are lucky enough to live without a chronic condition. I would argue that it's much scarier for the people actually living with it—but nevertheless, this concept of a possibly never-ending pain cycle is terrifying to some people. And in their attempt to comfort themselves that something like this could never happen to *them*, they end up projecting their "solutions" onto those of us living with the pain. I imagine it makes them feel better while making us feel worse. In their minds, something like this could *never* happen to them because they would take all the necessary steps to fix themselves. Those of us living in actual pain must just be missing something. We must not be trying hard enough.

I try not to be angry at those people (the ones who tell me to drink celery juice every morning, or go to a medical medium, or only eat plants and never touch sugar again, or fast every day for the next seven years) because I know that deep down, they're trying to help me. What I wish people understood, however, is that none of this is actually helpful. If it were that easy, I imagine I wouldn't be in pain anymore.

In the past, people have also implied that if I only had a more positive attitude then I might not be in so much pain. Beyond being rude as fuck to say to anyone, this also fails to understand the complexity of living with chronic pain and implies that it is simply a mental hurdle. I am not a weak person because I am sick. It is not because I couldn't find the positive in life, or because I don't see the glass as half full. I am sick because I have a disease in which tissue grows on my organs in places that it is not supposed to, causing me severe pain. If someone were positive and upbeat about this 24/7, I would be concerned. I no longer feel the need to lie and pretend that I feel positively about my illness 24/7, or that I feel optimistic about shoving a Valium suppository up my butthole every night in order to sleep for more than two hours at a time. Being honest and upfront about the very real limitations I experience because of my pain is not "being a pessimist." People are allowed to feel how they feel, myself included. It is not up to others to decide whether or not the emotions someone is experiencing are valid or not. No one on earth was appointed Gatekeeper of Valid Emotions.

I'm not sure why people's first instinct is to blame the person who is sick for being sick, but in my experience, it usually is. I can't imagine going up to someone who wears glasses and telling them their vision problems are probably just because they aren't eating a vegan diet and keeping a positive attitude, but crazier things have happened. As much as I wish my chronic pain were in my control, it isn't. And as much as people want to imply that it is somehow my fault that I am sick, it just isn't.

A large part of why this disbelief cuts so deep is that most people living with chronic illnesses, especially Vagina Problems, were told by doctors for years that the pain they felt was in their head. They made me feel like the pain I was experiencing was 1) fake or 2) somehow my fault. Because of this harmful messaging, when someone suggests a simple solution to my pain, or tells me to just "be more positive," I feel like they assume I'm sitting around day after day complaining that I'm in pain but doing absolutely nothing about it. Or it feels like they assume the pain is happening because of something I have done. If only I had not done the bad thing—like not going to yoga twenty-seven times a week—I probably would be just as healthy as Kelsey's cousin Jenna. And this is simply not true. One person may think, "Oh, I suggested a diet change because it made me feel better with the one health issue that I had, what's wrong with that?" And I get that. I do. *I DO.* I might have done the same prior to experiencing these illnesses myself. But now, instead of offering up unsolicited medical advice, ask yourself: "Did they ask for my advice?" If the answer is no, then for god's sake . . . please keep it to yourself. Rest assured, everyone, that if there were a simple or attainable solution to my chronic pain, I would have found it already. No one *wants* to be pain. I certainly do not.

I'm tired of the same rhetoric over and over again when it comes to chronic illnesses. We're not eating the right thing or doing the right medical treatment. We're trying too hard, or we're not trying hard enough. We're too sad, or we're in denial. No matter what it is, it's always our fault. I'm tired of people with chronic pain being blamed for being sick. It is not our fault. And no one with a chronic illness deserves to be in pain every day, no matter what they do or did, or what decisions they make.

* * *

I've begun to realize that people genuinely expect those of us with chronic pain to give up our whole lives just to *try* to feel normal. *Oh, you're still eating sugar when the majority of the world can with no consequences?? How dare you. Oh, you're still drinking alcohol on occasion even when you know it makes your pain flare worse? You must deserve to be in pain every day then! You mean to tell me you aren't doing yoga every single day? Not sure why you expect to be pain-free like the rest of the world then!* What people don't understand about having limitations around what we can and cannot do is that it's much more complicated than just changing up your diet or doing nine-teen stretches a day. It's not being able to enjoy simple things in life when it feels like everyone else can. There are many things that most able-bodied people participate in that those of us with chronic illnesses would be punished or judged for doing. If I go out to a bar on a Friday night and get drunk from two shots of Fireball and then have a bad pain day the next day, suddenly it's my fault and I'm not allowed to complain about it. I feel like I am in a constant battle between wanting to take care of my body while also desperately wanting to feel normal—or just like someone who isn't sick all the time. Like someone who can eat whatever they want without having to worry that one ingredient could upset their body so much that they spend four days in bed.

The reality of the situation, whether or not the general public likes it or agrees with it, is that I could give up sugar, or alcohol, or whatever the hell it is, for the rest of my life and still have bad pain days. Sugar may make *my* particular pain worse in some cases because it is inflammatory, yes, but it is not the *cause* of my pain—my chronic illnesses are. And when basically your entire life is dictated by an illness or illnesses that you have no control over, doing things that may cause you pain but **also** bring you joy is nearly impossible to avoid. Eating a cookie or going out on the weekend and having a glass of Moscato is like, *Hey, fuck you, illness! I can eat this cookie and I can go to this party and stay out late and you can't stop me!! I'm taking control of my life!!! I want to feel normal!!!!*

But then sometimes you pay for it, big time, and then it's a constant battle to decide which thing you want to deal with. Do I want to deal with missing my friend's party or do I want to deal with horrible pain down the line? Do I want to skip out on this team outing or do I want to order a pizza and share it with my friends and pretend to be a normal person without insane dietary restrictions? It's never an easy decision, and either way I'm left with regret. If I order the pizza, I'm mad at myself for knowingly doing something that could cause me pain. If I order nothing, I'm sad that it's yet another thing I have to give up or alter to accommodate an illness that I never asked for. When faced with these decisions, as minor as they are, I find myself feeling dejected all too often. Every bite of a cookie or missed social outing due to pain is a painful reminder (both physically and mentally) that I don't have control over my life, not really. If I said "fuck it" and did whatever I wanted, I would spend a lot of my life in bed with severe pain that wouldn't allow me to get up. But if I live a strict life and limit myself to things that will give me a chance of feeling better, I'm missing out anyway, and not living the life that I want to live.

It seems easy to people without pain, I imagine, to just give up everything in our lives that could make our pain worse. But it isn't. Those chocolate chip cookies I didn't eat start to represent every other part of life that I fear I miss out on because I'm sick. The pizza stands for the extra hours at work that I can't work because if I stay late, I won't function the next day. Those missed extra hours turn into the professional opportunities that I fear I have missed out on or will miss out on because I'm too busy resting after an exhausting day of just living my damn life. The wine represents the missed parties for friends or the missed date nights. It represents the vacation time spent in the hotel bed not sightseeing and the effort of trying to convince myself to remain positive. It should be easy to decide that I will no longer do things that could cause my physical pain to worsen. But like most things involving chronic pain, it's complicated. As I try to stop eating sugar and staying out late when I know I need sleep, I'm reminded that my life is not fully mine—not yet anyway. And that even when I strive hard to feel normal, or achieve the idea of normalcy that I cling so tightly to on my worst days, I am always different. It's a hard pill to swallow, one that would certainly feel easier if I could just take it with a chocolate chip cookie.

Despite how miserable my chronic pain makes me feel sometimes, I don't hate my life all the time. Or even most of the time. I recognize that as far as life goes, I am extremely lucky. And in terms of living with these particular chronic illnesses? I am privileged beyond belief. I have so much when others have so little. I am a thin white woman, which society has deemed acceptable. I do not have to experience additional bias—like fat bias or racial bias—when I go see a doctor. I can afford "alternative" treatment options like CBD, medical marijuana, acupuncture sessions, massages, and therapy. I have an understanding job that allows me to take sick days and work from home. I have a nice apartment and friends and family who are willing to come over and help me when I get really sick. But I am still in pain every single day. And knowing that it could always be worse does not, in fact, make chronic pain any easier to deal with. I have very few memories of the last decade of my life that are not impacted by my pain in some way. Birthday parties, weddings, dates, days at work—you name it, I have a memory tied to it that is filled with physical pain. And that really sucks.

But I think one of the things that bothers me most about living with chronic pain is the repetition of it all. I will have a particularly bad pain day, I will wallow, I will get angry, I will throw things, I will lose hours of my life and be forced to lie in bed. Then I will have to find some way to get through it, and to tell myself that it will end in due time. I will eventually get out of bed again, I will go back to work, I will go on walks. But then I'll have another bad pain day, and I will be forced to do it all over again. After more than a decade of this, it wears on me in ways that I cannot even find the words to describe. It is exhausting in every sense of the word to try to find a way to make peace with the knowledge that your own body will rebel against you, over and over again, and that there is essentially **nothing** you can do about it. It's the hardest pill I've ever had to swallow, and I have to swallow it again and again and again. It is like a giant horse pill that I am dry-swallowing with no water.

Living with chronic pain is not just being in pain. It's being forced to alter your life in a million different ways that other people don't have to, all while trying to find the mental capacity to be okay with this.

That's the other thing about chronic pain, and something I don't think is discussed nearly as much as it should be: the mental repercussions. As worn down as my body may feel sometimes, that fatigue almost pales in comparison to the way my mind feels. How do you find the strength and energy to enjoy little things in life when so many moments have been ripped away from you? How do you find it in you to care about the story your friend is telling you about their recent trip to Thailand when you were just forced to spend the last forty-eight hours in bed because you hurt so badly you were unable to walk? How do you find it in you to care about anything? How do you convince yourself to keep going when you know that if you do, you'll eventually be met with more pain? I don't always have the answer to this. I don't know how I keep going sometimes. There have been many days when I have not wanted to keep going. And there have also been many days when I have *not* kept going. When I've just stayed on my couch for twelve hours straight, not speaking to anyone. Not even watching television. Just sort of existing. And I think that's just it. I don't try as hard to find an answer anymore. I don't try as hard to push myself to stay positive or to tell myself it's going to be okay. Most of the time, I just try to let myself feel what I feel. Being able to admit my sadness, my anger, my frustration . . . all of it . . . is the only way I have found to make peace with this because I did not choose for my life to be defined this way.

People have asked me in the past what I wish people understood about living with Vagina Problems, or chronic pain in general. There are so many layers to it, but I think this is one thing that I most want people to understand: Having Vagina Problems does not just hinder my life during my period. It does not just hinder me when I try to have penetrative sex. It does not just come and go every once in a while, like a passing thought about getting Taco Bell for dinner. It is always there. It is always present. It is there when I get dressed in the morning and it is there when I sit down on a bench, or a desk chair, or a couch. It is there when I am at a wedding celebrating some of my closest friends, and it is also there when I am getting ready for bed each night. It does not ever go away—not really.

It seems like at least 80 percent of my life is just a waiting game. It's me waiting to see how bad the pain will be. Waiting to see if I'll have to cancel plans, or not leave bed, or consider an insane treatment option again. I sometimes feel like my life is all chronic pain with some living in between. I do my best to get through the bad pain days, hoping there will be a pain-free day on the other side. But once I get to that pain-free day, I'm simply waiting around again for the next bout of pain. People say the longer you wait for something, the more you appreciate it when it gets there. But with chronic pain, when the pain-free day finally arrives . . . you spend most of it worrying about when the pain will come back. It's a worry and a wait that never leaves you, no matter how many good pain days you have in a row. Because once you know what it feels like for your body to rebel against you, you don't forget it. And you spend most of your time trying to prevent it from happening again and worrying about when it undoubtedly will.

Normally I do my best to remind myself on these days of the positives. And I want to do the same today, in this book. But sometimes there aren't a lot of positives to living with chronic pain. Sometimes you just feel sad. And angry. And cheated. And that's okay. Honestly, it's okay if you feel like that a majority of the time. It's okay to let yourself feel. It's all part of the process. But in the same way that I wait for bad pain days—I'll also wait for the good. And I'll always remember that those days exist, too.

5

Why Won't Doctors Believe Us?

*I*t takes an average of seven years for a woman to be diagnosed with endometriosis, a disease that, as I have mentioned several times, affects one in ten women, or around two hundred million people worldwide. I continue to mention these statistics because it needs to be understood that one in ten women means it is not uncommon, and therefore it should not be this hard to receive a diagnosis. Endometriosis is, statistically speaking, as prevalent as diabetes in America—both affecting *at least* 10 percent of the population. But while diabetes is relatively easy to get a diagnosis for, endometriosis is not. Part of this is because to get an actual diagnosis for endometriosis, laparoscopic surgery is required. But a larger part of it is because we have a serious problem when it comes to doctors believing women's pain. And endometriosis is, inherently, a condition that only affects people with female anatomy. Seven years is a long time to wait for something that affects millions of people—and that diagnosis is only possible if the person living with it has the time, energy, and resources to see the number of doctors or specialists necessary to receive it.

It took me five years to get my own diagnosis, and I'm a thin white woman with enormous privilege in that I had the ability to see multiple doctors, was on my parents' decent medical insurance at the time, and am white. But I'm still a woman. And when it comes to women being believed in the medical world, we have a crisis.

I've often seen the question posed: "Is there gender bias in the medical community?" This question always makes me want to laugh. Not because it's funny, but because I can't believe people are still questioning this when it's not something that is up for debate, in my opinion. It's been shown in multiple studies that there is a clear gender bias when it comes to the way medical professionals treat women—especially women of color. I bet that if you ask any woman in your life if they've ever had an experience where they felt like the doctor dismissed their pain, you'd be hard-pressed to find someone who says no.

It's not just that women aren't listened to or heard when we go to our medical practitioners and tell them what we are experiencing, it's that there is also a very clear lack of funding and research dedicated to conditions that affect—you guessed it!—primarily women. A 2014 article in *The New York Times* titled "Health Researchers Will Get $10.1 Million to Counter Gender Bias in Studies" highlights part of this problem by explaining that women are rarely adequately represented in most clinical trials for new drugs or medical devices. But the gender bias starts before the drugs are even available to humans— many early studies work only with male lab animals, as scientists in the past have expressed worry that the hormonal cycles of female animals would skew results. One of the directors at the National Institutes of Health (NIH) was quoted in the article as saying, "We literally know less about every aspect of female biology compared to male biology." Great!!!!!!

Many doctors practicing Western medicine rely heavily on scientific studies and research when considering diagnoses or listening to explanations of symptoms. But studies and research for a majority of illnesses that affect people with female organs either don't exist or are few in number. Therefore, we are not only up against doctors blaming our symptoms on depression, or stress, or whatever dumb excuse they have for the day, we're also fighting against a system that has been in place for centuries now, which doesn't believe female anatomy deserves the same care and attention male anatomy does. All these things considered, it's not surprising that we hear so many stories from women about doctors dismissing their pain. But that certainly doesn't make it any more okay. How are the people living with endometriosis expected to fight back against the disease infiltrating their lives if they can't even find a doctor to believe that they have one?

* * *

I was fifteen years old the first time I passed out from my endometriosis pain. I was in the middle of doing wind sprints at basketball practice when the pain started. I told my coach I had to go and started sprinting toward the locker room. She scowled at me, thinking I was just trying to get out of wind sprints. I was really just trying to avoid vomiting on the hardwood floor. I somehow made it up the steps and into the girls' locker room before the pain exploded. I don't remember anything else right after that.

The next thing I do remember was seeing my coach, along

with some of my teammates. They were looking down at me, and the coach was on the phone with my mom. I was on the floor. My mom immediately got into her car and rushed to the school. By the time she got there, the pain had lessened to a dull ache. My mom asked if I wanted to go to the hospital. I told her we should just go to the urgent care center, if anything. She was worried, as any mother would be, but living in small-town Indiana, we weren't near many hospitals, and urgent care was closer. Plus, the thought of going to the emergency room scared me a little bit. So I agreed to go to urgent care.

When we arrived at the center forty-five minutes later, the excruciating pain I'd had in my stomach only an hour before had almost disappeared, leaving just an ache, like a reminder of what might happen again. When they finally called my name and took us back to a room, I was exhausted. I just wanted to go home. But I also wanted to know why the hell my stomach had hurt so bad. The doctor came in and sat across from my mother and me. The thing I remember distinctly about this interaction, above all else, was her refusal to direct questions to me. She only addressed my mother—as if she were the one who had passed out from pain. We began the usual routine of every doctor's visit I had ever made: *Give me your medical history. Has this ever happened before? Are you on any medications?* I answered all her questions, eagerly awaiting the part where she would tell me why I had passed out.

But before we could even dive into my symptoms, she paused. She was glancing at my letterman jacket, which was sitting beside me on the chair. She held up her hand to tell me to stop talking. I did.

What is that button on your jacket? Oh, that's a button in memory of my friend Emily. She passed away a couple of months ago and someone at school had them made. *Were you close to this girl?* Yes. I mean, she was my best friend. The doctor put her hand down and turned to my mom. *I see what the issue is here.* We both just looked at her, confused. What did my button remembering my friend Emily have to do with me passing out during basketball practice? She looked at my mom again and continued. *Your daughter is just sad, ma'am. I see this all the time. Something tragic happens in a young person's life and they act out to get attention. You should consider putting your daughter in therapy.*

I looked at my mom to make sure she was hearing the same thing I was hearing. She was wide-eyed and looked just as confused as I was. We sat in stunned silence, unsure if the doctor was being serious or dragging us along for some weird drawn-out joke. Then the doctor grabbed my jacket and held it up in front of my face. *You need to say goodbye to your friend, once and for all.*

I saw my reflection in my friend's face staring back at me from the button. I had bags under my eyes and looked exhausted. By this point, I was sure this doctor had lost her damn mind. Either that or this was all a dream and I was still unconscious on the floor of the girls' locker room. I looked at the doctor once more, confused and a little scared, but said nothing. *Go on, say your goodbye.*

It didn't seem like I had much of a choice. I wanted to get to the part where she figured out why my stomach kept hurting so badly. So I held on to my jacket, took the pin between my fingers, and said two words: *Goodbye, Emily.* The doctor wasn't satisfied and asked me to say it like I meant it. I wanted to get the hell away from her so I tried to make it sound more meaningful. *Goodbye, Emily, I will miss you.* It was bullshit, and I figured she would be able to tell. But she seemed satisfied and began to pack up her papers to leave the room. I kept thinking she might turn around and ask me more about my symptoms or order a test. But she didn't. She just left. And then my mom and I did too.

When I think back on this interaction now, years later, I wish I had said something more. I wish I had been able to explain to her that I knew very well what the pain of losing a loved one felt like—and it wasn't the pain I had felt in my stomach. I wish I had been able to at least describe my symptoms to her, or ask her questions about my pain, or demand a test be run. But I didn't do any of those things. I believed in doctors, I believed they had all the answers, and even though this one seemed a little outlandish, I assumed that everything must be fine. She wasn't worrying—so why should I?

I was eighteen the *first time* I briefly thought about checking myself into a mental institution. I was in college, and the pain I had experienced so often throughout my high school life was rearing its ugly head more and more often. I had just seen my gynecologist for the fourth time and, yet again, she could not give me a reason for the pain. She didn't even seem to believe me. Nearly every single day of my life my stomach hurt. I was swollen, constantly bloated, and always aching. But during my period, everything got much worse. I would throw up and lose consciousness. I had been forced to miss class and days of my internship. I would take pain pill after pain pill and find no relief. And my vagina? Yeah, it hurt. I had a lot of trouble trying to wear tampons, and it ached like a giant bruise more often than not. Sex was completely out of the question, but I wasn't even trying to have it anyway because I spent most of my time in bed, hugging a heating pad. I went through the usual with my gynecologist.

Are you taking birth control? Yes. *How long have you been on birth control now?* Since I was fourteen. *Do you take pain-killers around the time of your period?* Um, yes. So many that I'm not even sure it's safe anymore. *Hmm, maybe we will try a higher dose of ibuprofen.* I tried the 800-milligram ibuprofen last time, it didn't touch my pain, and it made me sick to my stomach. *You seem really upset. Are you stressed out? Stress definitely contributes to pain. Try to take some deep breaths.* I'm okay, I just don't know why this is happening to me. *It's normal to have some pain with your period. I'm more worried about your mental state. You seem to be suffering from some pretty extreme anxiety, which I think is contributing to your overall health.* Okay. I'm not trying to be upset. I'm just in pain all the time and I don't know why.

I had already tried taking her prescription-sized ibuprofen. It might as well have been a sugar pill. I even listened to the gastroenterologist's advice about food and was doing my best to follow a strict diet. I hadn't eaten gluten in weeks. This did nothing to ease my symptoms. The first time I saw this doctor, she brushed everything off and prescribed me a new birth control pill. The second time, prescription-strength ibuprofen. The third time, she mentioned trying to exercise more around the time of my flow. And this time she decided that I had heightened emotions, which might be contributing to the pain. She told me I was anxious and depressed. But it's pretty hard not to be when you are in serious pain for the majority of your life and your only source for answers isn't giving you any. Little did she know that I had already gone through my emo stage in high school, when I listened to Hawthorne Heights on repeat every day. I knew this wasn't just emotional. I was feeling real physical pain all over, but especially in my abdomen.

At first I thought it must be something with my stomach. I was visibly swollen and bloated in the stomach region

All. Of. The. Time. I had pain after eating, and I was pooping A LOT. Because so much of my pain resided in my abdomen, I assumed it had to be something involving my stomach. But I also had severely painful periods. Since I rarely paid attention during anatomy class, I didn't put two and two together that the pain might be coming from elsewhere.

It wasn't my job to memorize my old anatomy textbook and figure out the source of the intense pain I was experiencing, though. It was my doctors' job. And so far, all of them had failed me. Because I was so sure it was a stomach issue, I went to see two different gastroenterologists. Both told me to keep a food diary, and both concluded that my issues were due to "stress." Because of my painful periods, I ended up back in my gyne-cologist's office looking for answers. But she, like every other doctor I had seen thus far, gave me none. I left her office once again feeling hopeless and defeated, questioning my sanity. I went in knowing that my pain was real. But by the time I left, I wasn't so sure anymore. I went back to my dorm room and tried to ask a higher power to tell me what the hell was going on with my body. I begged for answers. *Please, God, Jesus, Buddha, anyone. Please tell me why this is happening and what I can do to stop it.* But no one answered.

I came to the conclusion that it must be in my head. Maybe I *was* depressed. And maybe I was just imagining it all. I began to convince myself that what I was feeling wasn't real. I con-tinued to do this for the next two years, every time I felt that familiar ache in my stomach. Was I just crazy? Should I be in an institution until I learned how to stop imagining this pain? But no matter how hard I tried to convince myself that the pain was a figment of my imagination, I never succeeded. And after a miserable and painful two years, when I ended up in the emergency room after passing out from severe abdominal pain (again), I stopped trying to convince myself.

I'll never forget that day. It was the week before Thanksgiving break. I was a junior in college, and I was trying to be more physically active. I thought the treadmill would be the place to start. (Honestly, fuck running. What I was thinking? But . . . moving on.) Two minutes into my run, I knew something was wrong. I started to feel that familiar cramping sensation in my stomach and got really scared. It meant that pain was coming. I pushed the emergency stop button on the treadmill and hopped off.

By the time my feet hit the floor, I could no longer stand up straight. The pain was severe, and it was getting worse. I doubled over and began crawling toward the bathroom. I knew I was going to vomit. I crawled into the bathroom, threw up in the closest stall, and then the pain *really* hit me. It shot through my abdomen, and I felt it in every single part of my body. I tried to breathe, but I became delirious. I was screaming, hoping that someone, anyone, would hear me. But I had been alone in the gym. I thought I was going to die. My phone had fallen on the floor next to me. I tried to reach for it to dial 911, but I no longer had control over my body; I was literally paralyzed. My hands were clenched so tightly from hyperventilation that I couldn't use my fingers to slide the unlock button on my iPhone, and I was in so much pain that I could not move from the ball I had curled myself into on the bathroom floor.

I tried and tried to get my phone unlocked, in between fits of screaming and trying to breathe. I knew I had to calm down and slow my breaths to regain use of my fingers and hands. But the pain was so severe, all I could do was scream. I once again thought I might die. I was desperate to call anyone. After what felt like twenty minutes, I managed to squeeze my paralyzed hands in the right direction and unlock my phone. I pressed on the most recent call on my phone, not caring who it was. It turned out to be my classmate Jenn. We had been working on a group project together the day before. Luckily I attended a small university and she was just five minutes' walk away. I don't even know how she understood me. She probably didn't. I just kept screaming that I was in the student center bathroom.

As close as she was, the time it took for her to get to me felt like years. I was in so much pain that I didn't even know how to breathe. It got so severe that I tried to hit my head hard enough on the toilet to knock myself out . . . but I couldn't lift myself enough off the floor to make an impact. I would have done anything in that moment to be free of the pain, but I couldn't even move. So I just waited and told myself that I wouldn't die. *Jenn is coming. Jenn is coming. This will be over soon. Breathe. You're alive. You can do this. You've done it before.*

I don't really remember Jenn coming into the bathroom, but clearly she did, and she called 911. The next thing I remember about that day is opening my eyes and seeing the student union pass me by as I was wheeled away on a stretcher. I ended up in an ambulance, where they immediately pumped me full of drugs. Next thing I knew, I was in the hospital, waiting to be seen by a doctor. I had high hopes about this doctor—after all, I had ended up in a fucking ambulance. I had to be taken seriously now, right? I dozed off again, and when I woke back up, my pain had lessened tremendously. I could breathe again.

I began to regain my consciousness and register where I

was. My dad was next to me. He had driven up to the hospital to meet me. Jenn was also there. She was rubbing my hand. It made me cry. The doctor came in and asked me to describe my symptoms. I did. This might go without saying, but it's really hard to describe extreme pain after the fact. You can tell someone "I passed out from the pain" or "I was literally delirious with pain" or "The pain was so bad I tried to hit my head on the toilet to knock myself out," but none of this means much to them unless they've experienced something similar. So while I did my best to tell my doctor exactly what I had been feeling, it didn't feel like I was doing it justice. How do you explain pain that overpowers your entire body without sounding like you're exaggerating?

I told him this wasn't the first time it had happened to me. I had passed out from my pain at least five times before—once at basketball practice; once in American Eagle Outfitters; once during an AAU basketball game; once when I was home alone; and once, after running around the cemetery in town, on my friend's living room floor. I told him how excruciating it had been and how scared I had been. I told him that I felt like I was going to die. I began to cry. And then I began to sob. I told him about how I had been having this mysterious abdominal pain for years now and how it would come when I least expected it and render me completely helpless. I told him how it scared me and how I just wanted to know what was wrong with me.

When I was finished, he barely reacted. He told me it sounded like severe period cramps. *Next time take Tylenol be-fore your period starts.* He didn't seem to register that I had told him four times that I wasn't even on my period. At this point you might be thinking, *Wait, no he didn't.* Unless you have endometriosis or you're a woman, of course; then you'll be thinking, *Wow, am I reading my own diary?* Yep, he fucking said that.

As he continued explaining that I should begin taking Tylenol three to four days before the start of my period, I began to question myself again. It was a habit at this point. *Had the pain really been that bad? How could it have been that bad if I was feeling better now? Was I dramatic? Was I making it up?* The doctor finished talking and I once again felt paralyzed, but this time it was mentally. I wanted answers so badly, but I had no idea how to ask for them. I had already tried.

But my dad hadn't. He pointed out again to the doctor that this wasn't the first time this had happened to me, and that I often complained of pain in my abdomen. Could it be my uterus? My ovaries? A stomach condition?

I felt around on your daughter's abdomen and felt nothing swollen or out of the ordinary. I really think your daughter just had period cramps that were a little more severe than she was used to.

I've never seen my dad look so angry . . . or shocked. He looked straight at the doctor and asked if he was going to do anything else to help me. It made me realize that maybe I should be shocked too. But I wasn't. If I had come to expect anything from doctors at that point, it was exactly what this doctor had done: suggest that my pain wasn't as bad as I said it was and deem it normal. And the Tylenol bit? Yeah, doctors seem to love suggesting over-the-counter painkillers to women who have endometriosis. Thank god for those doctors. Otherwise I might have never heard of the incredibly common and well-known painkiller called Tylenol. I might have never considered taking it either! I'd rather just be in pain, thanks!

I wish I could tell you that the doctor I saw in the ER the

night of my passing-out-while-trying-to-exercise fiasco was the last who treated me that way. But we both know I'd be lying. And I wish I could tell you that after that night I received a diagnosis and knew what was wrong with me. But, again, lie. By the time I actually received a full diagnosis, seven years had passed since my first episode of extreme pain and six months since Jenn called 911 for me. It was second semester of my junior year of college, and I had started dating someone.

At this point, I was twenty-one years old and had never *really* had sex. Partly because, as I mentioned, the one time I tried with my high school boyfriend had been excruciatingly painful, and partly because I was in pain all the time and rarely left bed. Also—have you met college boys? So when I started dating a boy in college, I decided to try sex. And boy let me tell you, it was hell.

Over the years, I've gotten better at trying to explain the pain of trying to insert anything into my vagina. So . . . let's try this out. Imagine you were going to insert a tampon, but it was the biggest tampon in the world, and your vagina was definitely not equipped to handle it. We're talking, like, the size of a rolled-up pair of socks. So you're trying to stick this big-ass tampon in your vagina, and it sucks. But WAIT, the tampon is now covered in acid. So now you gotta stick this giant thing in while it burns like crazy, and you feel as if your vagina is on fire. FUN, RIGHT? As you can probably guess, my attempt at being sexually active didn't end well. It lasted about forty-five seconds and ended with me screaming out in pain and him looking at me like I was crazy. He was visibly frustrated. *What is wrong with you?* Oh, how I wish I had known.

So I began googling again. I had googled my symptoms before, of course, but I never found anything that matched what I was experiencing, and I gave up pretty quickly when

I ended up on some websites that, naturally, told me I was probably dying. Getting back into it was scary, and I wasn't even sure where to begin. I had stomachaches a lot, but my vagina also hurt. Sex was painful. I could walk just fine, but sometimes as soon as I started to run, that severe pain would show the hell up again. It didn't really make sense, but I was desperately trying to save my relationship and hang on to any sense of normalcy I had left, so I googled.

And this time, I found something. I had been searching for several minutes and saw all the regular diagnoses: IBS, Crohn's disease, celiac disease, etc. It was all stuff I had been tested for, or things that didn't really match my symptoms. I decided to try something a little more specific . . . *extreme stomach pain when running.* I'll never forget the first time I saw the word "endometriosis." I had never heard of it or seen it before, so I clicked. It was accompanied by a list of symptoms. I had every single one. It even specifically mentioned severe abdominal pain while running, problems with digestion, pain after eating, and painful sex. I felt like Raven from *That's So Raven* when she's about to have a vision. Time stopped. Everything stood still. I began reading more about endometriosis and before I knew it, hours had passed. For the first time in more than five years, I actually wanted to go see a doctor. Armed with the information I had found on Google, I went to see a new gynecologist. This time it was someone I had known for years who was a well-known OB/GYN in the area that I lived in at the time. I had never seen him before because I had another gynecologist and didn't feel I needed to. But as things got worse, and I became more desperate, I figured he was a safe bet. I was optimistic for the first time in a long time.

It was a Thursday afternoon and I had just been called back by the nurse at my new gynecologist's office. She asked me the usual questions, and I didn't hesitate to give her honest answers. Before long the doctor came in. The appointment went great. I explained my symptoms to him and told him that I thought I had endometriosis. He agreed with me right away and told me that having a surgery could take care of my symptoms. JUST LIKE THAT!??! I decided that day to go through with the surgery and scheduled it for two weeks later. I barely even thought it through; I only thought of my life without the pain.

I never thought I would be excited to have a surgical procedure, but I was absolutely stoked to have this one. I truly believed that this would be what I needed to feel better—like it was that simple. I didn't even research the surgery, or bother getting a second opinion. After years of suffering, I just wanted to be pain free, and this surgery was supposed to do that. I also was about to leave for a semester to study abroad in Australia. It was my senior year of college, and I was going to fix myself! I was going to go to Australia pain free. Or so I thought.

Two weeks later, I went in for surgery. I kept thinking about how much my life would change. Looking back on it now, I don't even remember feeling nervous. Just excited. The surgery was early in the morning and both my parents went with me. The last thing I remember before going under is my doctor holding my hand and telling me he was going to fix me. I believed him. But he was wrong.

I try not to regret having the surgery. It gave me a long-awaited diagnosis. It started me on my path to figuring out what the hell was wrong with my body, and the path of armoring myself to fight back against it. But it also gave me more pain. Much more pain. At first, things were okay. Surgery had gone as planned. He had, indeed, found endometriosis, but assured me that he removed all traces of it. I had a diagnosis. I finally knew what was wrong with me, and I had a reason for the almost-constant pain I was feeling. I would be able to have pain-free sex! I would be able to eat foods without all that pain! I would be able to run! This was it. It was the end. *You'll start feeling better in no time,* he said.

Two weeks after my surgery, I left the country to study in Australia. It was supposed to be the time of my life. I was supposed to be free of my pain, free to live my life however I wanted to. It instead became four months of never-ending pain. A month into my time in Australia, the swelling in my abdomen that I had been experiencing for years somehow got even worse. The problems digesting became ten times worse. And on top that, if I thought my vagina hurt before the surgery, it was nothing compared to how it hurt after. It didn't take long for me to fall into a deep depression. I didn't understand what was going on. The surgery was supposed to fix me, so why was I feeling worse than before? I decided to reach out to my doctor.

Being in Australia meant that I had a fourteen-hour time difference with my doctor. I also didn't have a way to call a phone number in America without paying a pretty penny. My mother reached out to my doctor on my behalf and we were given an email address that I could use to communicate with him and his office while I was studying abroad.

I remember opening my computer to write the email to my doctor and immediately being overcome with emotion. I was lying in bed. My vagina was throbbing and my abdomen was so swollen that I had trouble taking deep breaths. I began to type.

Dear Dr. X,
How are you? I am doing okay, Australia is great. I just
wanted to reach out because I have been experiencing
some pain recently and I am a little worried. My abdomen
is incredibly swollen. It basically never goes away. I
have trouble wearing pants. And I'm still having a lot of
trouble with digesting food and eating without any pain
afterward. Is this normal? Is there anything I can do?

A couple of days later, while lying in bed in pain again, I
received a reply. I hurriedly clicked the email open, expecting
a solution or some sort of answer. Instead, I got this:

Hi Lara,
Dr. X said to tell you that it sounds like it might be what
you are eating. Are you drinking a lot of alcohol, as well?
Both can be contributing factors. Try to avoid alcohol as
much as you can and take some Miralax to help with the
abdominal bloat.

I wasn't sure how to feel. On one hand, I felt like I might
cry. On the other, I felt like I might throw my computer at
the wall until it broke into a million pieces. How could this
be happening again? As much as I didn't believe this doctor
or his advice about my eating habits, I was out of options. For
the next two weeks I was obsessive about the food I put into
my body. I ate the blandest food I could find, and I ate at very
strict times. But two weeks came and went and my abdominal
bloat only got worse. I was miserable. I spent as much time
as I could in Australia lying in bed with my heating pad and
wondering what the hell was wrong with me. It couldn't be
endometriosis, could it? He had removed that! I was supposed
to be feeling better. How could this be happening?

Three weeks after I sent my first email, I reached out again.

Hi Dr. X,
I took your advice and tried to change my eating habits.
Nothing helped, and I'm honestly feeling worse. I don't
know what to do anymore. I can't do this anymore. I'm
barely leaving bed. Any idea what could be going on?
Could it be something other than endometriosis? Any
ideas or advice is greatly appreciated.

It was a couple of days before I heard back with essentially
more of the same bullshit I had already heard. Try to get more
rest, eat bland foods, and try to calm yourself down. But there
was no calming me down. I had already gone through this
pain. That's why I had decided to have the surgery. This pain,
and this swelling, and all this shit was supposed to be in my
past. He had promised me I would be better. So why wasn't I?

Two months later I was back in the States and in the midst
of a dark depression. Any hope that I'd had prior to my surgery
had vanished completely.

I made an appointment to see my gynecologist. I thought
that maybe if we were able to talk in person, he would be able
to understand my symptoms a bit more and offer a solution.
He had been so understanding when I first went to him, prior
to my surgery. I thought he would be just as understanding
this time around. But he wasn't. Not even close. When I finally got to his office on a gloomy and cold January day, I
began to frantically describe my symptoms to him. I tried to
remain calm. I really did. But I had been bottling all this anxiety and fear for months. When I was finished describing all my
symptoms, I was sobbing. I could hardly breathe. He offered
me a Kleenex and told me he was concerned about the state of

my mental health. *You appear incredibly anxious with probable depression. Have you ever considered an antidepressant? It will also help with the pain symptoms you're describing.*

I had never tried an antidepressant. But I was willing to try anything. I left without any real answers and a prescription for antidepressants, which I filled that day and began taking religiously. The next two months were a blur. I was a zombie, a shell of my former self. I was in my second semester of my senior year of college and barely made it out of bed each day. I was missing days at a time of my internship and rarely going to class. I felt even more depressed than I had before starting the pills. I essentially lost my will to live. I was twenty-one years old, almost twenty-two, about to be a college graduate, and I couldn't imagine trying to hold down a full-time job, let alone getting out of bed every single day and socializing with people away from my heating pad.

I went back twice more to see my doctor. The first time, he upped my antidepressants to a stronger dose. The second time, he tested me for STDs after I told him that sex was even more excruciatingly painful than it had been before the surgery. I begged and pleaded for answers. I told him how low I felt, how hopeless I felt about my future. My feelings were dismissed and downplayed. I had nowhere else to turn, so I just gave up.

It would be another six months and a twelve-hour drive to the Mayo Clinic in Rochester, Minnesota—where I desperately turned when felt I had no options left—before I finally received a more in-depth diagnosis and an explanation for my pain. Yes, I had endometriosis. But I also had complete pelvic floor dysfunction and was given the diagnoses of vulvodynia, vaginismus, and vulvar vestibulitis. On top of the pelvic and vaginal pain I was experiencing, I had been operating under the notion that my endometriosis was gone. I was wrong. As it turned out, the surgery I'd had hadn't worked. All it had done was cause everything in my body that was already angry to become even more irate.

Currently, the most widely accepted and effective treatment for endometriosis is an excision surgery, where that tissue is removed by a surgeon. There are some pharmaceutical options available to suppress symptoms, but that is not the same as removing the endometriosis. Many top excision surgeons describe the pharmaceutical options as similar to putting a Band-Aid over a bullet hole. I did not have the excision surgery when I had my laparoscopic surgery mentioned above. I had an ablation surgery, which is when a surgeon uses a laser to burn off the tissue of endometriosis that they find. Although ablation surgery was widely thought to be effective for the treatment of endometriosis in the past, many experts now reject it because it only removes the top layer of tissue, meaning that most of the tissue is still there and will therefore still cause pain and symptoms. I did not know any of this when I opted to have that surgery in 2012. I did not know what endometriosis was, or what it meant to remove it. Most people do not. Many doctors don't even know the difference.

And it's not just that people don't know—it's also an accessibility issue. Up to this point, there has been no real distinction from the American College of Obstetricians and Gynecologists on the two surgeries and how the results of them vary greatly. Because of this, and because of the general lack of understanding when it comes to endometriosis and treatment of it, these two surgeries are considered the same to most insurance companies. But one of them—the gold-star treatment, excision surgery—requires a more specialized skill set and understanding of the disease and is therefore more expensive. When insurance companies see that a person with endometriosis wants to get excision surgery, they say, "Why can't you just get this ablation surgery that is thousands of dollars cheaper?" Therefore, excision surgery is often not covered by insurance—and that's if the surgeon even accepts insurance at all.

All my issues, all my pains were related. I did have endometriosis—which had in turn caused the onset of overall pelvic floor dysfunction, vaginismus, and vulvodynia. I also had probable adenomyosis—which is kind of like endometriosis, but is when cells similar to the endometrium are embedded in the muscular layers of the uterus.

It took the gynecologist at the Mayo Clinic less than five minutes to diagnose me with vulvodynia, a painful condition of the vagina. She then explained to me how all this was connected. It was a diagnosis and an answer that I had been waiting to hear for eight years.

I'll never get those eight years back. I will never be able to redo high school or go back and study abroad in Australia. All those days and nights I spent curled up in pain—those will never go away. And even after two full years of therapy, I still tend to minimize and question my pain because of what those doctors did. I often wonder if my past doctors ever think of me. I try not to think of them—but every time I have to go in for a routine checkup, I am forced to remember. My palms begin to sweat, my heart races, and I am on the defensive, prepared for them to question my every move. I want to forgive my doctors. I want to give them the benefit of the doubt, and I tell myself that they didn't know. I want to believe that they did the best they could. But their "best" ruined eight years of my life, and the answer was right there all along.

Fortunately I no longer need their validation. I now know what is wrong with me. I know that my pain is—and always has been—real. It's not a figment of my imagination, it's not a side effect of stress. It's real. The truth of the matter is, I don't even want my doctors' remorse. I don't want an apology. I just want change. I want doctors to do better. I want them to listen to women, believe women, and help women. After all, our pain is real. And we won't stop fighting until you finally believe us.

6

Hi, My Vagina Hurts, Wanna Date?

*I*t was a Tuesday night and I was sitting on my bed, staring at myself in my full-length mirror while I wrapped pieces of my hair around a curling wand. I was twenty-two years old and living in Los Angeles. Although it was mid-April, the evening was hot, and the Hollywood apartment I had moved into after arriving in Los Angeles just three months prior didn't have air conditioning. My every attempt to get my hair to lie in loose, effortless curls was failing miserably. I put the curling wand down on the floor and looked at myself in the mirror. I was wearing my blue dress from ASOS—the one I had bought on a whim when I found out I would be moving to Los Angeles. It was sticking to my thighs. I could feel my nerves deep in my stomach; they were clenched so tightly I could hardly breathe. My neck was drenched in sweat, and my hands were clammy. I tried to take deep breaths, but they weren't doing much to unclench the muscles in my stomach. I grabbed my phone, which was next to me on the bed, and began to type.

I'm so sorry, I know this is so last minute, but my car just busted a tire and I'm not going to be able to make it tonight . . .

Hey—I'm really sorry but I can't make it tonight. Hope you understand.

Heyyyy! Any way we can reschedule? Work is so crazy today, I can't get away.

I typed and deleted and typed again for fifteen minutes. I didn't send any of them. I put my phone in my purse to prevent myself from pressing send. I had ten minutes before I had to leave, or I would be late. My hands were shaking as I tried to run my fingers through my hair and give it some volume. I looked at myself in the mirror once more and noticed the sweat on my brow. My lips were dry, my eyes wide. *It's just coffee*, I told myself. Just. Coffee. With a boy. Who would probably, at some point, want to have sex with me. And I knew that might never happen. I tried to imagine how the date would go, and how I might casually slip my secret into conversation.

Yeah, haha, and by the way, I might never be able to have sex with you. But I'm still pretty funny and I can make decent banana bread.

Yeah, interesting that you mentioned the one time you were sick. I actually have this illness that kind of never goes away? And it makes my vagina hurt, like, a lot. Anyway, do you wanna split an appetizer?

Every scenario I could think of only made my stomach clench tighter. I'm not sure how I got my legs to work and pull me up from my bed, down my stairs, and toward my car, but I did. And there I was, driving to get coffee with a boy who had no idea that my vagina had . . . a lot of problems. He ordered us both a beer and a coffee. The date was off to a horrible start—drinking caffeine or alcohol of any kind usually gives me bladder pain that lasts for twenty-four to forty-eight hours. I ordered water on the side and decided to sip the beer. It seemed easier than trying to explain why a twenty-two-year-old didn't drink coffee *or* alcohol. But then again, maybe that was the opening I needed.

Yeah, I'm actually not drinking this beer because I have a chronic illness and also, I can't have sex with you, haha. Anyway, where did you say you worked again?

We talked about the usual things—his work, my work, where we grew up, and his dog. I nodded when I was supposed to and laughed on cue, all while thinking about what it might be like to tell him that I might not ever be able to have penetrative sex with him. The date didn't last very long, and when he made a move to leave, I jumped at the opportunity. He offered to walk me to my car, but I politely declined and practically ran from the cafe. By the time I got to my car, I had tears pouring down my face. I was exhausted, even though we had barely spent two hours together. How was I going to do this the rest of my life? How was I going to continue on date after date until I (hopefully) found someone who was understanding? And even if I could do that, how was I ever going to be able to explain my problem? And if I could explain it, how would I ever find someone who accepted it—truly accepted it? It had only been one date, just over two hours of my life, but I was already sick of dating. I knew I wouldn't hear from him again, and although I thought I might be sad, I mostly just felt relief.

* * *

I had dated prior to this—if you want to call it that—but I was in college. My only other relationship experiences up to that point had been the guy I called my boyfriend on and off from seventh grade until high school, and since we couldn't even go on real dates for 90 percent of our relationship, that hardly prepared me for the Los Angeles dating scene of my future. We also didn't have sex. We tried to, once, but it was a disaster and lasted all of five seconds because, spoiler alert, it fucking hurt.

Everyone told me my first time was supposed to hurt. It's like some unwritten rule—I grew up knowing that whenever I chose to have sex for the first time, it would hurt. But I didn't expect it to hurt *that* bad. (And by the way, SEX SHOULDN'T FUCKING HURT, even your first time.) After that experience I basically avoided dating and physical contact with the opposite sex until college. And that's when I started to realize just how many problems my vagina actually had.

I was twenty years old, a junior in college, and trying desperately to fit in and feel some sense of normalcy. And there he was, twenty-one years old, an athlete, and someone I had known prior to college. I thought he was a safe bet. It started out relatively normal—lots of texting, and making him wait two hours before I responded to appear busier than I actually was. And I guess at first it *was* normal. Until we tried to have sex.

It was our third attempt and it was going just as badly as the first two times. I was staring up at the ceiling, and I could feel the tears start to escape from my eyes. He was on top of me, missionary position, and thrusting into me over and over again. It didn't feel good. In fact, it hurt so badly I was biting my lip to keep from yelling out. But although I was counting down the seconds until it was over, he somehow seemed to be enjoying himself. So I let him continue. I thought maybe, in time, it would get better for me. I thought maybe I would be able to enjoy it too. I thought this was somehow what was supposed to be happening.

He climaxed and rolled off me. I tried to hide the sigh of relief I felt escape from my mouth. I pulled up his jersey cotton sheet, which had never been washed, to cover my body as I tried to slow my breath and contain my tears. I could feel him looking at me, but I didn't want to meet his eyes. I wanted to run from the room. I wanted to teleport to my own dorm room and get under the covers and never come out again. But I also wanted him to hug me, to kiss my forehead, or grab my hand like he used to, or wrap me in his arms and tell me that everything would be okay. *What's wrong with you*, he asked instead. *This keeps happening.* I didn't have an answer. I wanted to say something, but what could I say? I didn't know what was wrong. I didn't know why this kept happening. I didn't have an answer for anything. So I stayed silent.

He eventually rolled over and grabbed his boxers off the floor. He put them on and then went into his bathroom and turned on the shower. I heard the water and the shower curtain move. I started to unravel as the tears came faster. I sat up and frantically looked for my own clothing. I pulled my underwear, sweatshirt, sweatpants, and socks on; grabbed my phone; and left the room. When I got back to my dorm I collapsed into my bed and let myself cry. What *was* wrong with me? I wish I knew.

As you can probably imagine, based on the fact that I dedicated an entire chapter of this book to dating with Vagina Problems, the men in my life have not exactly been understanding when it comes to these issues. And College Athlete Boy wasn't an exception.

In his defense (though I am well aware he doesn't necessarily deserve one), I wasn't equipped to explain it to him. I would freak out, and my body would start to involuntarily shake, and I had no explanation for it. Sex was fucking painful, but I didn't know why. *I* didn't even know what was going on with my body, so how could I explain it to *him?* It's not like I was sitting him down over dinner, bringing up my Vagina Problems, and offering up a solid explanation. I was undiagnosed at the time. I had no idea that these conditions were even a thing! So my solution for dealing with the awkwardness and the whole me-screaming-out-in-pain-during-sex thing was to mumble my apologies and insist that I was working on getting it fixed. That is . . . when I wasn't turning away from him to cry and ignoring him completely. And look, I know that everyone talks shit about their exes, but seriously, he was not great at dealing with this.

Looking back on it now, I know that it wasn't exactly an ideal situation for either of us. And there are layers to this shit. There always are. But the idea of sex between heterosexuals has constantly been reinforced as the act of a penis going into a vagina until the man gets off. And that's basically it. I didn't even know women *could* get off from penetrative sex until I was well into college, and even then, that knowledge paired with what I experienced during sex didn't leave me optimistic. So yes, I was very visibly in pain, both mentally and physically, and he would just encourage me to push through the pain so he could get off. And yes, he never once comforted me after we attempted to have sex. In fact, he actually looked annoyed when I would cry from the pain, and he would leave as soon as he could. That, or he would immediately jump in the shower and leave me in his twin bed with my Victoria's Secret PINK underwear discarded to the side while I tried to figure out what the hell had just happened.

Although our sexual encounters were awkward, unenjoyable (for me), and full of confusion, we continued seeing each other for a few months. I suppose that, in his mind, sex was supposed to be his penis in my vagina, with the end result of him ejaculating, and that was what was happening. And although to me it was *very fucking obvious* that I was in pain and not enjoying it, who the hell knows what he thought was going on? (Like I said, I know he doesn't deserve my defense, and I'm not sure why I feel compelled to give it to him. I sometimes still fantasize about being in that dorm room and pushing him off of me and telling him that he's a fucking prick, screaming at him that men who don't go down on women definitely won't be getting into heaven.) But I can also look back now, five-plus years later and with lots of therapy under my belt, and realize that maybe he didn't know what to do. Maybe he was scared! Maybe I wasn't communicating what the fuck was happening and not providing an opening for a conversation about it. He was confused, I am sure. And for that, I give him 12 percent of my sympathy. Because guess what? As confused as he might have been, so was I. And I was the one dealing with the actual fucking pain.

* * *

If you can't believe that I saw College Athlete Boy for months, don't worry. I can't either. And honestly, I can't believe he continued to see me. What was either of us getting out of it? Surely he wasn't dying to find a girl to watch him watch *How I Met Your Mother*? And lord knows I certainly wasn't dying to find a guy who I could sit next to while he watched a show that I didn't even enjoy.

But one thing that is crucial to understand about having Vagina Problems, which I most definitely did not understand at age twenty, is that they have a special way of making you believe you are unlovable. When I was seeing this guy, I fully believed that being loved by someone was synonymous with having a sexual relationship with them. And I believed this because it was what I had been told time and time again by TV shows, commercials, magazines, and movies.

Seeing as how I spent so much time in bed during my college years due to unexplained pain, I watched my fair share of TV. TV told me that sex was vital to any relationship. And it wasn't just TV, it was everything. I saw it in movies, I read it in magazines, I heard it from my friends, and it was implied in every shitty joke about marriage that I had ever heard. *HAHA, who wants to get married, right??? Having less sex over the years?? NO THANKS.* Sex was *everywhere.* And since I couldn't have it, at least not in the way that I felt was expected of me at the time, I believed that no one would ever want to be with me, and no one would ever be able to love me. I felt broken and incomplete.

So when I found someone (like College Athlete Boy) who (sort of, barely) seemed to accept me despite my shortcomings in the bedroom, I felt like I had to put up with everything he did because it had to be better than being alone. Up until the point of attempting to sleep with College Athlete Boy, I had managed to suppress and ignore most of my feelings about the pain related to sex I had experienced. This was in part because my sexual experiences prior to college were so limited, and also in part because I didn't have an outlet to talk about it. That's not to say that I didn't have supportive friends or family members in my life—I did. But even so, trying to talk about something so intimate, embarrassing, personal, and confusing is not easy. *Hey, so, when you guys are, like, having sex, haha, with your boyfriend or whatever . . . do you, like, scream out in pain?* It took me literally YEARS to even open up to my best friends about what was happening to me, and it certainly wasn't while I was in college.

When I did finally tell friends about it, years later, I didn't even speak the words aloud. I wrote about it, because writing seemed easier than trying to speak the words into existence— that my vagina hurt so badly that I could not stand for a man to touch it, that I could not wear underwear, or jeans, or sit down for long periods of time. And if I didn't feel comfortable opening up to my closest friends in college or right after—the same friends I was pooping in front of and puking in front of after drinking too much cheap vodka at a house party—then how the hell was I supposed to tell a man I was romantically interested in? Let alone tell a doctor? The same doctors who had, for years at this point, been reinforcing the idea that the pain I was feeling was *not real?*

Attempting to have sex at this stage in my life with College Athlete Boy, or be sexual in any way, while still experiencing such intense, real, physical pain, finally forced me to face my pain head on. Because every time I attempted sex, I could no longer ignore it. I could no longer pretend that this pain didn't affect every single part of my life. It was there, smacking me in the face, reminding me day after day that something was going on in my body. I just didn't know what. The more disappointed looks I saw from College Athlete Boy, and the more he asked me what was wrong with me, the more determined I became to figure it out.

* * *

Before we go on, there's one thing about my Vagina Problems that has to be communicated. That is: It isn't only insertion that causes me pain. Just getting aroused can cause a shooting pain from my pelvic area throughout my entire body. It feels like what I imagine getting seventeen bee stings and a period cramp all at the same time would feel like. All those muscles are clenched so tightly, and they are so accustomed to being in pain, that they simply rebel and fight back. It's as if they are saying to me, "Bitch, what the FUCK ARE YOU DOING????" It can feel as if I'm being punished. It's not exactly an aphrodisiac. In order to continue experimenting and ~get frisky~ I oftentimes have to push through a certain amount of pain and determine just how badly I want to try. And anyone touching my vagina? In the year 2012? Before I knew about pelvic floor physical therapy? Before I had heard of a dilator? Nope, no fucking way. I couldn't even touch my own vagina at the time. Underwear couldn't touch my vagina.

My vagina was constantly on edge. It needed Xanax, a deep-tissue massage, and a really, really good therapist. After years of painful and less-than-comfortable gynecologist exams, followed by years of painful sexual experiences in college and thereafter that seemingly had no explanation, I could hardly blame it. No one was getting near that thing without my body reacting in a negative way. No matter how hard I tried, how much I wanted it, how much wine I drank or how many pep talks I gave myself, my entire body would begin to shake if a man so much as caressed my lower back. I would begin to sweat, and I flinched like crazy. I had zero control over it. Fooling around wasn't usually a fun experience for me. I had always had a certain sense of dread when it came to the idea of fooling around with someone. Forget touching my vagina, GOOD LUCK EVEN TOUCHING MY FOREARM.

Despite this, I still wanted to experiment and attempt to be intimate because a) I felt like I had to in order to feel a sense of normalcy and b) I wanted to do whatever I wanted to do, my body be damned!

Of course, I've seen the comments online on essentially every piece I have ever written that mentions my pain related to sex. I've been a writer on the internet for more than six years now, and I've written about my pain a lot since college, so that's a lot of comments. Yes, I know I shouldn't read the comments. But I did. I do. I still do. *Just do anal. Your mouth still works. It's called lube. This girl sounds like a nutcase. Seems like it's all in her head. She should see a psychologist. You have more than one hole for a reason!* I've had people say to me, literally more times than I will ever be able to count, *Dude, just don't have sex.* But anyone who thinks this fails to understand what it's like to have such a basic part of life stripped away from you.

I have never once in my life, to this day, had an experience with traditional penis-in-the-vagina sex that didn't leave me curled up in mind-boggling pain for hours afterward. I've never once been able to orgasm without *some sort of pain shooting through my body.* Although it's gotten less severe recently due to the years of work I put in with dilators, pelvic floor physical therapy, and experiments on my own time, I still, to this day, cannot orgasm without some sort of side effect. I've never even been able to become aroused without some inkling of pain! And if my body thinks I've orgasmed too many times, I get punished for that too. But guess what, it's not 1887, and women want sex too! I'm allowed to want to get off. *I WANT TO ORGASM.*

So despite my experience with College Athlete Boy, and

despite eventually receiving diagnoses that came with no cure and little hope that my vagina would get better anytime soon, I continued to try to experiment and fool around because I wanted to! And even though it hurt me time and time again in different ways, I continued to try to find a way to make it work for me because I felt like I needed that in my life. During a time when everything felt out of my control, the work I could put in at physical therapy and at home with my dilators felt like something that I could *maybe* control. I couldn't control the endometriosis that was seemingly spreading throughout my organs causing me daily pain, and I couldn't control the way my legs felt after walking on hard pavement because of my pelvic floor issues. But the more work I put in with physical therapy, the more I realized I could potentially have control over orgasming and sexual experiences. And I needed that. Not only did I need it, I wanted it.

* * *

It was a Thursday morning and I was lying on my back with my left knee bent and my left foot resting against my right leg. My physical therapist had one hand inside my vagina and the other hand on my abdomen. I had been in pelvic floor physical therapy in Los Angeles on and off for four years at this point, and I had made *a lot* of progress. Though I was still unable to have penetrative sex, a fact that my brain reminded me of every time I started to feel optimistic, I was orgasming with less intense pain, and orgasming more often. At age twenty-seven, I had discovered the art of using a vibrator just two years prior and had been trying to use it every day for the previous six months or so.

"When I first started to see you, you weren't able to handle this level of insertion from my finger at all." I looked up at my physical therapist and felt myself smile. She was right. And while my brain had been focusing on the fact that a finger inside my vagina was still painful, I reminded myself to celebrate the small stuff. It had been a long journey. A journey that I was, in many ways, still on.

"Have you gone on any more dates recently?"

I felt my body tense. She felt it too. I broke my eye contact with her and looked to the side. "It's just really hard. Even though I know there are lots of different ways to have sex, it doesn't make telling someone any easier."

I was single again, after recently getting out of a three-year relationship. I was once again navigating the dating scene with my Vagina Problems, but this time I was four years older and seemingly wiser.

* * *

They say that practice makes perfect. But I'd been practicing telling men about my Vagina Problems for the last six months or so, and I wasn't sure it was getting any easier. In fact, sometimes it actually felt like it was somehow getting harder. Although being in a long-term relationship where I did not have penetrative sex helped me realize that a sex life is very much still possible without penetration, it was still hard for me to see myself as someone who could be desirable to someone else long-term. Regardless of how much progress I'd made in talking about my pain—and I'd made A LOT over the previous four years—it still never felt easy to disclose this part of my life. People ask me all the time: When is the right time to tell someone? And I'd tried each option: telling someone right away via texting in a dating app; telling them in person on our first date; letting them know when we decided to become intimate by blurting it out right as they were kissing my neck; or not saying anything at all and running out of the bedroom crying with no explanation after we started getting physical.

As much as I hate to say it, there is no correct answer here. There's no easy or surefire way to tell someone about this stuff. I don't think it's ever going to feel like the right time because it will always feel like boiling-hot water burning your tongue after you spit it out. Your stomach will feel tight, your hands will clench in your lap. If you're face-to-face, you'll do your best to avoid eye contact because you don't want to see that look. You know the look I mean. The one you've seen time and time again that translates to, "Jesus Christ, I gotta get out of here." If you're texting it or communicating about it over some other technology, you'll hide your phone under a pillow and feel like you're going to faint, puke, or both until you see their name light up on your screen with a reply. You'll want to read it right away, but also never want to read it at all. You try not to overanalyze anything that is said or done regardless of how it comes out because you know that even the most well-intentioned people can fuck up when talking about Vagina Problems.

What I have come to realize, after forcing myself to continue dating and putting myself out there, is that there is no right way to tell someone. There just isn't. There's no magic time for letting someone know. The only rule that you should follow is telling someone whenever the hell you feel ready. Whenever you feel comfortable and ready to share that part of your life with them, tell them. If you don't feel ready, then don't. Ryan from Bumble isn't showing up at this bar and sitting across from you and immediately telling you about his deep-rooted issues with his absent father that can cause him to have trouble trying to get close to someone. Most people do not go on dates and throw all their baggage out there for the other person to sort through and decide whether or not they can handle it right away. We don't have to either.

I used to share because I felt like I had to. It felt as if I were keeping a secret from my dates if I didn't let them know up front. I shared this with my therapist once, and she asked me why. "Why do you think you owe them this explanation before you even know if you like them?" I thought long and hard about it. Why *was* I sharing this info with people so quickly? Why did Jeff from Hinge get to know intimate details about the way in which I was able to have sex before I even knew his middle name? I vowed to stop doing this. But trying to stop, after more than five years of doing it, was like my attempt at quitting sugar cold turkey. It was fucking hard. I had to start by identifying the ways in which I presented my Vagina Problems as a huge, daunting secret—one that I felt obligated to share with all my dates immediately. Every time I caught myself wanting to tell them up front, or apologize prematurely, I had to resist the urge. It was like resisting a gooey, warm chocolate chip cookie from Subway when I was two days away from starting my period.

I did my best to retrain my brain so that when I felt the urge to apologize, the words would feel like acid on my tongue. Reminding myself of what my therapist said helped. It was like a mantra that I began repeating to myself: *He is trying to impress you too. You don't owe him an explanation. He hasn't earned one yet. He has shit too! Everyone does! Yours isn't any worse than anyone else's! It's just different!* Jake, the dude sitting across the table from me at the bar, is not some fucking god who doesn't have any trauma. If we're being honest, Jake probably has more baggage than I do. Jake has probably never seen a therapist and will get too drunk and tell me about the girl who cheated on him when he was seventeen years old. He's thirty-two now, but he's still not over it. Sure, my vagina hurts and therefore I can't have a penis inside me, but at least I'm not thirty-two years old and still unable to deal with someone cheating on me when I was seventeen. Perspective.

Oftentimes, divulging to potential lovers has been a defense mechanism. Depending on how they reacted, I would know if they were worth my time. I've encountered enough shitty men along the way to know that some people really aren't okay with Vagina Problems. Some people do not and will not want to deal with them. And that's okay. I mean, it fucking hurts. It feels like someone is ripping my heart out of my chest each time. It certainly takes a toll on my self-esteem. It can make me feel like I never wanna go on another fucking date again. But genuinely, it's okay. Because realistically, if someone cannot be compassionate and kind about something that causes me great pain—both physically and emotionally—up front, then the chances of that person being a good fit for me long-term are slim to none. And the chances of that person being even close to deserving of seeing my vagina are pretty low. And by pretty low, I mean I should never show those people my vagina. They don't deserve it. But telling myself that doesn't make it hurt any less.

So yes, telling people quickly and up front about my Vagina Problems has been my unintentional way of trying to weed those people out. I don't want to get to know someone over five dates and develop feelings for them only to have them rip my heart from my chest and spit on it when I find out they're not cool with what I have going on. I'd rather know up front.

The strategy of blurting out your shit early on is both good and bad. It's good because sometimes it really does weed people out. It can get rid of the Kyles who don't give a shit about your hopes and dreams and only care about where they can stick their penis, saving you a lot of time and energy that could be better spent elsewhere. But it can also be bad. I think sometimes people with Vagina Problems, or a chronic illness of any kind, have a habit of deciding how people will feel about dealing with the problem without actually giving them a chance to form their own opinion or show us how they feel. I certainly do this. It keeps bad people away, sure. But it can also keep good people away.

Personally, I am now so used to the idea of people turning away from my pain or seeing it as a burden or an annoyance that when faced with someone who maybe doesn't view things this way, I don't believe it. I assume they just don't understand the full scale of the situation. Maybe they're naive about what is actually happening—maybe they don't fully grasp what I'm saying. Like, no, Justin, it's not just tonight that I can't have penetrative sex with you. It's a thing that I'm honestly not sure will ever go away.

And if you somehow manage to get past the painful sex part, how do you approach the shit storm that is living with a chronic illness as a whole? If someone somehow manages to say they're cool with that, I absolutely assume they just don't understand me. Maybe they didn't hear me because a car drove by, maybe they were distracted by thoughts of an upcoming work project—whatever it is, they certainly couldn't have heard me. And if they did, they must not grasp how often I actually do have to spend a day in bed, or how much my illnesses do affect me every day. When I start to think about that and remember the way people have handled it in the past, I begin to panic. And I start throwing more stuff their way.

"Lara, it's okay. You're sick. I understand. I don't hold that against you. I hope you feel better soon, and we can reschedule. I'll text you tomorrow."

"Okay, but I might not feel better tomorrow. Because it's not a flu. I don't have a cold. I have a chronic illness. I might have to miss our next date too! Who knows! I never know how I am going to feel! It's completely unpredictable!! And this is only the tip of the iceberg!! We haven't even gotten into a relationship together yet!! We've only gone on a few dates!! What if we continue to see each other and then I can't even make it to your birthday party? Did you know I've had to miss *my own birthday* for the last three years due to pain??"

I keep throwing additional things at them, almost as if I'm trying to convince them they should stay away. And maybe I am. Because deep down, there's a part of me that has been convinced of that very thing—that people *should* stay away. It's a self-destructive pattern, and one I've only started to identify in the last year or so. It's also a defense mechanism, much like telling people quickly and up front—and it's a successful one. For the most part, it's subconscious; I don't even realize I'm doing it until the person on the receiving end of my shit-tossing takes a step back and says, "Woah, what is going on here?" I then tell myself, "Well, you knew this was going to happen!" and move on, leaving them written in my past as just another person who couldn't accept me.

But did I *know* it was going to happen? Or did I take steps that contributed to it happening?

For a long time, when a man I was dating failed to meet my needs, I would internalize it, thinking I was too much, or that I was the problem. This rhetoric has been pushed on me a lot in past relationships. I was always asking for too much. I talked about my pain too much. I used it as an excuse. I was impossible to deal with. Blah. Blah. Blah. So much so that sometimes when I even mention that I'm having a bad pain day, or have a doctor's appointment, or that I'm even "writing a book about my vagina" to someone I'm romantically interested in, I can feel sweat start to form on the back of my neck. My chest starts to tighten, and I start downplaying what's going on, or backtracking on what I was trying to reveal. *Haha, yeah, I live with a debilitating chronic illness that causes me a lot of pain, but don't worry! I'm still a ~fun~ and ~cool~ girl who just may never be able to, you know, have your dick inside me! But I'm totally fine with it. It's fine. See, I'm smiling. Don't you believe me?* I feel the need to make others comfortable with a situation that I'm definitely not comfortable with myself. And when they aren't equipped to deal with it or understand the full scale of what I'm facing on any given day, I find myself once again preparing to accept defeat and tell myself that I knew this was going to happen—that who I am and the way I function . . . it's just too much to deal with.

But with a lot of therapy, repetition of my daily mantra about who I am and what the fuck I deserve, and a lot of time spent on the couch, crying into my dog's fur, I have started to realize something that I still have to remind myself of daily: It's not at all that *I* am too much. Maybe these people just weren't enough for me. Maybe they aren't worth my time and energy. I think letting anyone in my life, and this goes for anyone with a chronic illness (especially Vagina Problems), requires that they possess a certain level of empathy and understanding. I had to stop going into dates worrying about what these people would think of *me and my issues,* and instead ask myself what *I* felt about *them and their issues.* Because everyone has them. Everyone. I can't settle for the Justins or Nicks of the world who say things like, "Ugh, it just sucks. I, like, really wanna have sex with you, though." If the only way you can figure out how to have sex with me, you fucking dingus, is to stick your penis in me, then I'm 1,000 percent sure I don't wanna have sex with you anyway!

I try not to feel guilty or badly about this because, ultimately, every person on earth requires different care or has needs of some kind. The kind I require isn't better or worse—it's just different. And not everyone will be able to give me what I want or need in relationships.

So I continue going on dates. Both because I want to, and because I think it's good for me—healthy, even. For a long time I was so ashamed of my pain and the effect it had on my life that I couldn't even speak to a man I found attractive. It took years of work to get to the place where I'm not only comfortable speaking about my pain, I'm also not ashamed of it anymore. It took an almost insurmountable amount of work—work that I am still doing every day—to get to a place where I still feel attractive in this body, or like I could be desirable in any way even though I am often in pain, especially sexually. Now, for the most part, I no longer feel like it's something I have to apologize for. I no longer believe that men who date me "despite" my conditions are "doing me a favor." I do my best to accept what I have and remind myself that it doesn't make me any less worthy of love, affection, or intimacy. What I have is just what I have. And everyone has something.

Over the years I have done *a lot* to try to make it possible for me to be sexually active. As soon as I got my diagnoses in 2012 and 2013, I began pelvic floor physical therapy and started doing my best to insert vaginal dilators every single day. I used ice packs on my vagina and used a machine to pulse all my pelvic floor muscles to help them relax. I tried coconut oil, yoga, meditation, acupuncture, chiropractic work, deep-tissue massages, and a bunch of self-help books. I took about eighteen vitamins and supplements a day and avoided all thong-style underwear. I changed my laundry detergent and bought more loose-fitting pants and skirts. I even tried putting chili cream on my vagina at one point.

Some of it helped, most of it didn't. But the thing that ultimately helped me the most was reframing the way I thought about sex in general. What was sex? What *is* sex? As I mentioned, for most of my teen and adult years, my idea of sex had simply been a penis in a vagina. And therefore, because of my conditions, I thought of sex as something I couldn't do. Even the way I talked about sex—whether it be with potential partners or friends, or when I wrote about it online—it was the same wording: "I can't have sex."

But the truth of the matter is that I *can* have sex. I just can't currently have penetrative sex. And, as I mentioned earlier, that is just a teeny tiny part of what sex actually is or can be. I'm absolutely not going to sit here, writing this damn book, and pretend that reaching a point where I understood sex as more than just a penis in a vagina was easy. It took years. YEARS of work. But once I realized that I could very much still have a sex life if I wanted one, and that there was a whole world of opportunity out there, I gave myself permission to start seeing myself as someone who could be desirable again.

* * *

"Do you wanna get out of here and go back to my place?" I asked. The music had gotten louder, and I could barely hear myself think. It was a Saturday night and we'd been sitting at my go-to bar for first dates for an hour and a half. The conversation had flowed easily. I had made a small dent in my vodka water with lime—a drink that I had only recently discovered left me in less pain than other mixed drinks—and he was on his third whiskey ginger. His hand was casually resting on my knee, and for once I didn't feel sweat start to form on the back of my neck. Instead, I leaned into his touch and did my best to maintain eye contact and give him my flirty smile.

I was twenty-seven years old and was once again back on the dating scene in Los Angeles. He was twenty-nine, six foot three, and very much *my type*. He had shaggy blond hair that looked as if it hadn't been washed in days while smelling like it had been washed only hours before we met up. He wore a plain white T-shirt with navy blue Dickies pants and Vans. We had talked for a couple of days on Hinge before agreeing to meet on this night. He was a subpar texter—I wasn't laughing out loud at his texts or spending hours rereading our conversations by any means—but I enjoyed it nonetheless. He was confident, and made it clear he was into me. As the conversation continued and his hand moved closer to my thigh, I felt myself leaning into it more and more. I wanted this. He wanted this.

"Let's go," he said. We got in an Uber and went to my place. I was slightly tipsy, in the best way, and was laughing easily. There was a brief moment, in the back of that Uber, where I wondered how he would react when he found out that we would not be having penetrative sex. But as quickly as that thought entered my mind, I shoved it out. This was fun. I was enjoying myself. And I wasn't going to entertain those thoughts right now. Not yet.

The Uber pulled up next to my building and we both hopped out. As we walked up to the front door, his hand caressed the small of my back. By the time we got inside, I was shaking. But for once, it wasn't necessarily because I was scared. I was excited. We sat on my couch and shared a joint—in part because I knew it would help my pain levels, and in part because I knew it would make us both feel a bit more relaxed. We watched clips on YouTube and laughed together. And then, suddenly, his mouth was on mine. He tasted like whiskey and ginger and I couldn't get enough.

After we made out on my couch for a while, I stood up and asked him to come back to my bedroom. I felt alive . . . and exhilarated. I didn't feel like myself, while also feeling like the most powerful version of myself. It was like I was role-playing, or watching this unfold from somewhere else. As we began undressing, I asked him if he wanted to borrow some pajamas. He laughed, which made me laugh because my matching two-piece set from Target was certainly not going to fit him. Whether it was the easy laughter, the weed, or the half of a vodka water I drank, I began feeling more and more at ease. I lay down next to him and, as things began to progress further, I blurted it out. "I don't do penetration."

He stopped kissing my neck for a second and peered up at me, waiting for me to say more. I continued, "It just can hurt me because of this illness I have. I can do oral and other stuff, though." I did my best to say it as nonchalantly as possible, just like I had practiced in my mirror mere hours prior. I felt an apology start to rise in my throat and immediately pushed it back down. *You are not sorry. You are owning this. Do not apologize.* He started kissing my neck again. "That's cool with me. If I do anything that causes you pain, will you tell me?" I nodded and felt my body release tension I didn't know it was keeping as I fully relaxed into his touch.

I orgasmed five times over the course of the next eight hours, and the next morning, when I watched him from my bedroom window get in his Uber and leave, tears started pouring down my face. This time I wasn't sad, though. This time I was crying because I had finally done it. I had experienced a sexual encounter that did not leave me feeling less than, or like I needed to apologize. I spent the rest of the day in my leopard robe, crying tears of happiness on and off as I realized just how far I'd come.

*   *   *

It was hard—and is still sometimes difficult—for me not to believe that my Vagina Problems are a deal breaker when it comes to dating. That the way they sometimes make me behave, or the pain they so often cause in my life, is absolutely the reason that so many of my past relationships have not worked. It doesn't matter if it's a long-term relationship or someone I've just dated a couple of times—if they suddenly disappear, I always assume it's because of my illnesses. It's hard not to feel like a burden. It's hard not to have this idea that I'm forcing my partner to miss out on having a relationship with someone who is "whole."

Because anyone living with this shit knows that it's not just living with pain, it's also not being able to do certain things. And it's not just not being able to do certain things—it's having extreme anxiety, sometimes depression, and walls so high you couldn't scale them if you tried for days. It's not a single-layer issue that will go away after one failed attempt at having sex. It's not one discussion where you say, "Hey, I have some vaginal pain, but it's cool," and then move on from it forever. It's ten thousand moments and maybe just as many conversations about it and the ways it impacts your life and relationships. But that still doesn't make it a deal breaker.

The thing is, I don't want to be this way. I don't want to have the physical pain. But I especially don't want to have the emotional baggage that comes hand in hand with it. No one wants to be this way. I don't want to be so guarded or terrified of letting people in. But like anyone who has been burned in relationships, that's so much easier said than done. I told myself a thousand times that my Vagina Problems didn't make me unlovable, yet I didn't really believe it until the last nine months or so—and that's even after my ex-partner of more than three years told me that they weren't a deal breaker. I can and will continue to tell myself, and anyone else with Vagina Problems, a thousand times a day if I have to, that this stuff, these problems—they don't make us less desirable or harder to love. In the past, it meant less to me coming from myself. And I hate that. I want to believe that the way I am, the way I work and the way I don't—it's all fine, it's acceptable, and it doesn't make me any less deserving of love. And on many levels, I *do* believe that. I'm a goddamn catch—vaginal pain or not! But I won't pretend that it's been easy—or that it is easy now.

The world does not yet embrace people with Vagina Problems. Men's erectile dysfunction has been recognized and given treatment options for decades now, and I'm still hard-pressed to find a doctor who even believes that my vaginal pain is real—or that it deserves attention and care from the medical industry. Yet, despite all the shit stacked against us, those of us with Vagina Problems don't have to continue to stay quiet or believe that the only way we are able to work is wrong in some way. Whether or not society—and, more importantly, the medical industry—ever recognizes how detrimental living with Vagina Problems can be to someone's entire life isn't up to me. But I'll make damn sure they keep hearing about it.

No doctor ever gave me permission to say, "Sex is painful for me and I am allowed to be upset about that fact." But after years and years of trying to find a way to live with this shit, I gave myself permission. And I'm giving you permission, too. I am allowed to want to have sex simply for pleasure. I deserve that just as much as any other human being on this planet. I do not have to stay silent about my pain just because it is misunderstood, or because it is considered taboo to talk about. I do not care if talking about my vaginal pain is uncomfortable for other people because no matter what, it will always be more uncomfortable for me . . . the person living with it.

Once I gave myself permission to feel these things in general, it became easier to transfer the method over into my dating practice. The thing that absolutely, hands down helped me the most on my dating journey was learning how to stop apologizing and start owning what is going on with my body.

What I am sure of now, more than ever before, is that I am so much more than the way my vagina does or does not work. And so are you. There is so much more to dating, relationships, and life in general than having sex. If you're dating someone worthy of your time—you will figure it out. Because where there is a will, there is a way. I no longer approach dates feeling as if they are doing me a favor. I don't ask myself if they're going to want to keep seeing me once they "find out" that I can't have penetrative sex. I only worry about whether or not the person I am spending time with is someone I actually want to spend time with. The rest of the stuff? I can figure it out later.

7

Love, Lust, and Vagina Problems

When I first decided that I wanted to try to write this book, I was in a long-term relationship. We had begun dating at the end of 2014, after being friends for some time. By the time I began working on the proposal for what is now this very book, we had been together for more than three years. We lived together. We adopted a dog together. We went on family vacations and took pictures for Christmas cards. I thought we were in it for the long haul. I thought I had it all figured out. So when I wrote my book proposal and outlined the chapters I wanted to write, I knew I wanted to include one about being in a relationship with Vagina Problems. As someone who had not always been in a relationship and had been on the dating scene with this stuff, I knew how hard it could be to imagine that a man would actually want to be in a long-term relationship with someone who not only couldn't have penetrative sex, but who also dealt with almost daily pain. I wanted to instill hope in everyone reading this book who had not yet found a loving and understanding partner that it *was* possible. But as I sit here writing this chapter now, a year after that relationship fell apart, I know that all I was really doing was trying to convince *myself* of those very things. I wanted to believe that the relationship I was in was my happily ever after. But it was not.

Most of the memories I have from growing up and fantasizing about love and relationships revolve around the belief that love is effortless. I always thought that when you love someone, really love them, nothing else matters. Sometimes that love will be tested; should difficulties arise in a relationship, then one person, or both, will wonder if those difficulties are too much for them and contemplate leaving the relationship. Maybe one person is closed off emotionally due to being hurt in the past. Or maybe the other is so accustomed to being on their own that they just don't know how to function as a pair. Or perhaps one of them has some sort of baggage—weird family, depression, whatever it may be—and runs away from the other person because they are scared. Things get tense. The future of the relationship is suddenly in question. But then, at the last second, one or both people will realize that love can conquer whatever the problem is, and then they will run to each other and embrace. Weird family, commitment issues— whatever the problem is, it falls to the wayside. Just like that. You have one discussion, one argument, one fight . . . and it's figured out. Forever.

When I was first diagnosed with Vagina Problems and began contemplating what it could mean for my love life, I spent a lot of time dreaming about finding love. Even before I had a word for what was happening in that region of my body, it still prevented me from being intimate or opening up to men emotionally in ways that could eventually lead to a love connection. But I wanted it. I wanted it so badly. I would sit in my one-bedroom apartment in Carmel, Indiana, just months after graduating college, and stare at my eggshell-white living room wall with the scent of a Bath & Body Works candle burning in the distance, and I would fantasize about what love would look like for me.

It was always a variation of the same vision, over and over again: me telling a man that I loved that I would not be able to do something, like sex, or go somewhere, like dinner, because I was in too much pain. Then him sitting down next to me on the bed or the couch, telling me that he understood. He would push my hair behind my ear, kiss my forehead, and settle in on the couch or bed with me while we waited for the worst of the pain to pass. We would spend the time in between my bouts of pain laughing, embracing, and knowing that everything would be okay. It was everything I had seen in movies and TV shows over the years, but with the addition of my Vagina Problems. It was a man telling me that he didn't care whether or not his penis could go inside of me on this day or any other—and actually meaning it.

I craved this acceptance so badly. It was a fixture in my thoughts for the entire year after I was given my diagnosis of vaginismus and other pelvic floor problems. I just wanted someone—a man that I cared for—to tell me that it was okay. That I was okay. That the way I functioned was okay. And that he still loved me despite it.

As the years passed and I moved out to Los Angeles, my fantasy altered a bit. It became a picture in my mind of the two of us—me and this mystery man I was hopelessly in love with—driving off into the sunset on the Pacific Coast Highway, on our way to Malibu. He would be driving, I would be in the passenger seat, sitting cross-legged because that's the most comfortable position for me with my pelvic floor issues. His hand would be resting gently on my thigh. I wouldn't feel a pit in my stomach at the hint of an intimate touch, but instead I would lean into it, because he would know all about my pain, my fears, my anxieties—and he would accept them. We would ride off into the sunset together and never have to worry about my Vagina Problems again. It wouldn't feel like a burden, or like a giant elephant sitting in the car with us. It wouldn't even be an issue. It was a different scene, but the idea remained. I craved acceptance so badly I could taste it. Love, to me, meant finding a man who saw my sickness and didn't run away from it.

This fantasy of love with my Vagina Problems worked for a little bit, until I tried to apply it to my real life. When I eventually met someone, my now ex-partner, and entered into a long-term relationship a year or so after moving out to Los Angeles, I tried desperately to make that fantasy of love with Vagina Problems become a reality. But despite my attempts at making my relationship into the perfect fantasy I had always dreamt of . . . it wasn't that easy. The first couple of times that I had to miss events, or shy away from intimacy, or spend twelve hours in bed, depressed, thinking about my future with pain because I was unable to walk, I was generally met with understanding and compassion. "Lara, it's no big deal, let's just order Thai food and watch *The Sopranos*," he would say. It was the thirty-fifth or the seventy-fifth time that I had to do this, however, when things began to fall apart. That's what they don't show you in the movies or on TV. They don't show you what it's like to live with something that is chronic—meaning it doesn't go away after you solve it the first time. It doesn't even go away after you talk about it—at length—for the seventy-fifth time or the three hundred thirty-eighth time. It is still there, lingering, messing shit up. And that's just one of the things that makes love with Vagina Problems so damn hard sometimes.

As our relationship grew, so did my pain. But what grew more than anything was my anxiety around my pain. It became difficult for me to leave the house. Half the time it was because I was actually *in pain*, but the other half was because I was sure the pain would appear at any moment. During this time, I began to see myself as some sort of giant monster. I felt as if I were two different people. There is the relationship with Lara, and then there is the relationship with Lara who is in pain. And that Lara . . . well, she's a monster. She is like the Beast from *Beauty and the Beast*, but without the giant mansion. I think of this Lara—Lara who is in pain—as a nightmare to be around. I am a tornado, destroying any place I set foot in and leaving a massive mess to clean up in my wake. Because of my pain, I demand attention and require extra care. I can be mean, I sometimes lash out, and no one, not even my partner, wants to be around me. I am always sad; I bring down the mood. I am unrelenting, just like the pain in my body.

I miss things. I miss out on friends' birthdays, memories, picking up on social cues, small talk, you name it . . . I've missed it while in pain. And I sometimes cause my partner to miss things with me. I am always in need of something from my partner—whether that be attention, a heating pad, a joint to smoke, taking my dog for a walk because I can't, bringing me a glass of water because I find my legs are unable to work, or just being there when I am in pain once again and having a hard time dealing with it. I'm needy.

It's hard to imagine myself as a human being when I get like this. It's easier to imagine myself as a big monster wrecking everything. Because that's what it feels like inside my body—everything is a mess. But beyond seeing myself as a monster, or a tornado destroying everything in its path, or a giant burden to everyone in my life, what it really comes down to is this: I see myself as unlovable.

Unlovable. That word has haunted me for years. It seems foolish now, on my good days, to think that there have been so many times in my life where I have truly believed, with everything in me, that the person I am is not worth loving. Years of therapy have taught me that this belief stems from various moments in my life including—but not limited to—past relationships and the media/society's portrayal of what love is. But when you have a steady stream of relationships that don't work out, and you also have chronic pain that inhibits you from being sexually active in a way that is expected of straight women, it's hard not to believe that the reason your relationships continue to fail is because of those problems. And the constant messaging about what love is that I was fed growing up by all my beloved TV shows and movies—well, it's hardly what I would call an accurate portrayal.

Love is, as it turns out, not easy. It is not meeting someone that you fancy and agreeing to spend the rest of your lives together, with no issues. It is not making it through one difficult situation and figuring it out forever. Love is constant work. It is not only working together but working on yourselves, separately. It is existing as a unit while also finding a way to remain independent. I believe that love will always be worth it. But it won't be easy.

I hated who I was when I was in pain. I hated everything about it. I hated the way it made me feel—both physically and mentally. I despised the way my stomach swelled at my waist when I looked in the mirror, as if my uterus were fighting to leave my body behind. I hated the way my clothes fit or rubbed against my vulva in a way that brought tears to my eyes and nausea to my stomach. I no longer enjoyed eating because every bite of food would cause inflammation, making my body feel as if a thousand red fire ants were gnawing on every inch of my skin. I hated the mess my pain seemed to cause. Clothes strung out over the floor because I couldn't find anything to wear and had no energy to put any of the discarded items away in drawers. Crumbs of food covering the living room floor from me dragging the only food I could find that sounded remotely edible with me to the couch in an attempt to keep my body nourished.

But more than anything, I hated the way my partner reacted to my pain. He would refer to me as cold or tell me that I didn't smile when I didn't feel well. He would distance himself from me when I experienced a bad pain flare. He said he never knew how I would react. I guess I didn't either. To me, everything felt hard. In some ways, everything *was* hard. But my anxiety and depression made everything that much harder. It was a constant battle—not necessarily between my partner and me, but between me and myself. I would enter another pain cycle and do my best to get through it, but then the bad mood and anger would begin to swell inside me. And from there, I began spiraling.

I reprimanded myself constantly. In my mind, I was never doing enough. Sure, I was in extreme pain. But did I have to just sit on the couch crying about it? Why couldn't I just be a better partner and go to our mutual friend's party with him? Yes, I was sick. But did I have to *act* this fucking sick all the time? The reprimanding wasn't fair to myself. Maybe how I acted when in pain sometimes wasn't fair to him either. But in a relationship when one person is sick and the other is not, it rarely ever feels *fair*. I had no one to blame but the illnesses inside my body, and when that stopped being enough, I began to blame myself.

I knew that my partner and I were struggling. I knew that we were no longer connecting in the way we had when we first started dating. But instead of facing that head on, I hid behind my pain in many ways. Every time we had a disagreement or a big blowout fight, I would tell myself it was because I was so hard to deal with. *You just have a short fuse because you don't feel well. We're not enjoying each other's company as much anymore because you aren't enjoying much of anything.* I told myself that all the problems we had could be traced back to the fact that I was sick. Not only that I was sick, but that the way in which I handled my illnesses made me difficult to be with. I was a burden. I was asking for too much. And my partner? Well, he didn't disagree with me.

I had so much hatred and anger for the pain in my body that seemed to be wrecking every area of my life that it was easy for me to blame the demise of my relationship on this pain as well. After all, if I weren't in pain and miserable more than 50 percent of the time, *would* we be fighting? Would we have any problems at all? I wasn't sure. Blaming all our problems on my pain felt easier than facing the reality, which was that maybe we just weren't a good match for each other. Blaming my pain felt good. I was angry, but being angry didn't make me feel any better, so I propelled that anger into blame. It didn't make the situation feel any better, but I needed something to blame. And I was so tired of blaming myself.

In many, many ways, I had become dependent on my partner. He was my security blanket. Even when we were fighting, or unhappy, or barely hanging on to the semblance of a relationship, I craved being around him. I felt like I needed him. Knowing that he was there gave me a sense of comfort. *If I pass out from my pain today, at least he will be here. If I have nothing else in this life because it has been taken away from me by this disease, at least I still have him.* He stopped being a person I was in a relationship with and instead became a symbol of whether or not I was lovable. As long as I had him and the relationship, I believed I had to be lovable. At least in some way. It stopped being about finding that great love for me, and it became only about being in a relationship simply to prove to myself that I could be—even with my pain.

Because it was so hard to see myself as someone worth being in a relationship with, when I did begin dating my ex-partner, instead of searching for someone who truly met all my needs, I was only searching for someone who would accept me. I didn't ask for more than that. I didn't ask for anything else—because I didn't believe I deserved anything else. If he was going to take on the burden of spending part of his life with me . . . then that should be enough, right? But it wasn't. Of course it wasn't. I didn't ask for butterflies in my stomach or for unwavering support even on my worst days. I didn't ask for spontaneity or a connection so deep that you felt sure the two of you were destined to meet . . . you just had to be. All I asked for was love. I didn't specify what kind. I didn't specify for how long. I didn't indicate how I wanted this love to be shown to me. I just wanted to be loved. Period. Point blank.

When my relationship eventually ended in the summer of 2018, after three and a half years together, I forgot how to breathe. It felt like the entire world stopped moving. Everything was in slow motion while I was spinning wildly out of control. I sat in my apartment—the apartment we had shared together—in the dark, with the curtains closed, and watched as he packed away his things and dismantled the life we had built together. I sat on my couch in my snot-covered forest-green nightgown and looked around me at the apartment we had moved into together less than a year before. I saw the marks on the floor from our shoes when we played chase with Pepper together. I noticed a crumb on the coffee table from the last time we ordered Popeye's chicken on DoorDash after a long day at work. He was everywhere. We were everywhere in that apartment. Everywhere I looked I was bombarded with another memory. Eventually, I had to close my eyes. But sleep did not come. I just sat there, like a zombie. For three days I did not eat. I did not sleep. I did not shower or leave my apartment. I cried. A lot. And while he moved all his belongings into our guest bedroom until he found a place of his own, I got on my knees and begged and begged for him to change his mind about us.

I was overcome with a sadness that felt as if it would never leave me. The next day, as I once again sat on the couch we had picked out together at Crate & Barrel a mere nine months before, I saw that fantasy about love with Vagina Problems that I had had all those years ago drift further and further away in my mind. I no longer felt like I knew how to function on my own. What was I going to do? The same thoughts kept turning over and over in my head. *How would I ever find someone else? If he didn't love me, how would anyone else? This is it. This is how the rest of my life is going to be. This is what I deserve for being so hard to love.* I blamed myself entirely for the demise of the relationship. Not only did I blame myself, but I *hated* myself for it. I hated my body and the illnesses inside of it. I hated that it felt like my illnesses, and my pain, had won—that they had finally proven to me after all those years that maybe those voices in my head were right all along. Maybe I was unlovable.

In retrospect, those thoughts were how I should have known that we were not a fit. When the relationship finally came to an end, most of what I thought about wasn't how much I would miss him, but how much I feared being on my own. And how much I feared once again being a single person with Vagina Problems. I wasn't positive that I would miss waking up next to him every morning or spending our weekends together—the last year or so of our relationship had been tumultuous at best; it was difficult for us to be around each other at all, let alone continue to live together in a committed relationship. But instead of thinking of that, or acknowledging the bit of relief I felt somewhere deep down at not being in the relationship anymore, the only thing I could focus on was that I had just lost the only person who would ever choose to date me despite knowing I was sick. It felt as if my worst fear had come true: I was unlovable.

My entire self-worth had been tied up in this relationship. So naturally, when it ended . . . I questioned my self-worth even more than before. If the person who lived with me for the better part of two and a half years couldn't understand the complexities of my pain and help me navigate it instead of turning away from it, how would anyone? If this person, the person to whom I pledged my love and vice versa, could only last a mere three and a half years dealing with it, how could I expect anyone to last a lifetime? I kept going back to the idea of what I wanted love to be like for me. I thought I had found it. Maybe I did find it, for a little bit. But in finding it, I discovered that it wasn't actually what I was searching for. I was looking for more. I just didn't believe I deserved it.

Like most people who have gone through a breakup, there's certainly been a part of me that has wanted to talk shit about my ex at one point or another. And while I could easily do that here right now, and say that he was horrible, at times, dealing with my illnesses, and that he made me feel like even more of a burden than I already do, it would be completely unfair to not also acknowledge what this relationship did for me. It was not the right fit, yes, and it lasted much longer than it should have, but it gave me the foundation I needed to begin to change the way that I thought about love with Vagina Problems.

Going into this relationship, and other relationships I have had in the past, I always assumed that my inability to be sexual in the way that was expected of me, or in the way that I wanted to be, would surely be the demise of the relationship. I anticipated that when my relationships inevitably came to an end that I would absolutely know the reason why—and the reason would be that I wasn't able to have penetrative sex. But I was wrong, and this relationship showed me that.

At the end of this relationship, there was no part of me that could blame my inability to have penetrative sex for the end of our relationship. I tried to place the blame there. I did my best to tell myself over and over again that if I only had a working body, we'd still be together. But even when I told myself these things, no part of me really believed it. My ex-partner and I had a sex life. We were intimate in ways that I had not been intimate with other people. There were many points during our relationship where I honestly forgot that I wasn't able to have penetration, or a "normal sex life," because it was such a nonfactor. Not being able to have his penis inside me was not the reason our relationship ended. It wasn't even close.

For us, it was as if I could not eat peanuts because I was allergic. I told him that, early on, and he never asked me to eat peanuts again. In fact, he never even hinted at it. And honestly, why would he? If you care enough about someone to enter into a committed relationship with them, and you know that peanuts cause them pain, why in the hell would you want your partner to eat them? You wouldn't. Even if you really, really loved peanuts—like, they were your favorite snack of all time—you would get rid of the peanuts in your house and start stocking your shelves with other options, like macadamia nuts or cashews. That is what we did with our sex life. (I never thought I would compare a sex life to having cashews in your pantry, but I do like cashews quite a bit, so here we are.)

If nothing else, this relationship taught me that when you care for someone, when you really care for them, you will figure it out. Because when it comes down to it, every couple has their own version of sex. Everyone has different wants and needs, so no two sex lives are alike. Intimacy is how you express desire, pleasure, love, and lust to someone you care about. You can be intimate however you want to be. Limiting this to just penetrative sex does a disservice to us all. This relationship didn't work out, but with time and reconsideration of what the relationship actually was, it reassured me that future relationships might—despite my Vagina Problems. I just have to remember to throw out the peanuts and stock the shelves with lots of cashews.

Stephen Chbosky once said, *We accept the love we think we deserve.* What kind of love does someone like me deserve? The answer, of course, is unconditional and fulfilling just like anyone else. But that's not the answer I gave myself. And it's not the answer I always give myself in the present day either. The truth is, I could write ten thousand words trying to convince myself and anyone else who lives with Vagina Problems that we are just as worthy of love and intimacy and everything we could hope and wish for in romantic relationships as anyone else, but the belief has to come from within. It's not something you can say to yourself once and hope it sinks in. It's not even something you can say to yourself for a week straight and hope it eventually sticks in your brain forever. For me, it's a constant practice. And one that I am still practicing daily.

These days, when I envision that great love with my Vagina Problems that I fantasized about all those years ago, the concept has changed quite a bit. I still want love despite my pain, yes, but I also want more than that. And not only do I *want* more than that, I know now that I *deserve* more than that. I want someone who sees my pain as a strength, not a weakness. I want someone who embraces the idea of staying in on a Saturday night and getting high on the couch because my uterus hurts too much to do anything else. It wouldn't feel like missing out on adventures, because the two of us spending time on the couch together *would be* the adventure. I want someone who is open and willing to explore an intimate and sexual relationship in twenty thousand different ways and never feel as if they're missing out on anything because of my inability to do certain things. I want someone who doesn't shy away from me when I am in pain, but thinks it's cute and charming when I get mad at my microwave for taking too long to heat up my rice-filled heating pad. I want someone who brings me water and walks my dog for me not because I beg him to do so when I can't get up myself, but because he sees that I am struggling and he wants to help me.

I don't want to feel the urge to hide my pain, or my sadness, or my anger around my person. I want to just be me and know that despite everything, who I am is more than enough. I still want to ride off into the sunset on the Pacific Coast Highway with someone, but that someone has to offer me more than just love. Above all else, I want to get to the place where I know that even if I never find this great love that I've always dreamt of . . . it doesn't mean anything. It doesn't make me unlovable or unworthy of affection. I am existing in the only way I am able. And that in itself is enough. It will always be enough.

I sometimes still struggle with the idea of being unlovable. It's usually during a bad pain day, when I start down the familiar path of wondering why anyone would ever want to spend their life with me. Although the voice inside my head that tells me I am not good enough the way I am is now often dormant, it has not disappeared. I'm not sure it ever will entirely. But instead of focusing on making it go away, I now allow myself to focus on not listening to it anymore. I will not lie to you and tell you that I am 100 percent at the place where I see my worth and will never settle for less than I deserve in a relationship again. But I am closer than I have ever been before. And that—much like the person I am despite my Vagina Problems—is enough.

8

My Friends Constantly Talk About Their Sex Lives,
and I'm Trying Not to Hate Them:
How to Remain Friends with People
Who Don't Have Vagina Problems

My friends and I were in Palm Springs to celebrate my twenty-eighth birthday. We had decided to forgo leaving our Airbnb for the weekend and instead went grocery shopping to have enough food on hand for every meal. Saturday night we were going to make tacos—with a special bowl for me to fit all my dietary restrictions. I was on day five of my period by the time we made it to the Airbnb. I was barely bleeding, and I felt pretty good. The week following my period is usually one of the only relatively easy pain weeks I have in any given month. I was optimistic. I brought weed with me to Palm Springs, since medical marijuana is the only form of pain management I am currently using, but I didn't pack my usual bag of trinkets in case of a bad pain flare. I assumed I would be okay. After all, it was only a weekend. And the only plans we had for the weekend were swimming, eating, sleeping, and taking scandalous Instagram pictures.

On Saturday afternoon, after a long day of swimming and lounging topless, I decided to take a long nap. I had consumed quite a bit of CBD, which left me feeling slightly drowsy. I took a shower and crawled naked into my crisp, white Airbnb bed. When I woke up two hours later, I was feeling pretty good. Good enough, in fact, that when my friend opened a bottle of prosecco and asked me if I wanted a glass, I said, "Hell yes I do." I made it through half a glass before the pain started. It came on slowly, and then all at once. At first it felt like relatively normal bladder pain—the kind I deal with all the time. Like an aching and burning in my abdomen, similar to the pain you may feel after holding your pee in for too long during an Avengers movie. But before long, it turned into something else entirely. In a matter of twenty minutes I went from sitting on the couch in the Airbnb waiting for the moment when we all got hungry enough to start making tacos, to lying sideways, to eventually curling myself in a tight ball so I could more easily squeeze my abdomen. It was starting to hurt, and it was starting to hurt bad.

I could feel the fear start to rise in my stomach and make its way to my chest. My hands felt clammy and the hairs on the back of my neck were prickling. I told myself to remain calm. I went through all the usual affirmations I say to myself every time, whether they help or not. *You are going to be okay. This is going to pass. Just breathe. Stay still. The more upset you become, the worse the pain will be. Breathe. Breathe. Breathe.*

I could hear as my friends started chopping the onions and peppers for the tacos in the next room. The noise sounded oddly far away, even though I was mere feet away. The pots and pans were clinking. I knew I should get up and help. I wanted to call out and ask if there was anything I could do, any vegetables that I could chop, but no sound came out when I opened my mouth. I briefly thought about going to my bedroom to grab my heating pad. Knowing it might be my only window of opportunity, I pulled myself off the couch and crawled to the bedroom. I assumed that once I plugged in the heating pad and got some weed in my system, I would start feeling better.

I was wrong. I put my heating pad on its highest setting, wrapped it around my abdomen, and pressed it into myself as tightly as I could. I found a joint and took three hits. It hurt so fucking bad. Tears started pouring down my face as I curled myself into a ball on the couch again and tried to focus on the television in the background. *Below Deck* was on. It was one of my favorite shows, but I couldn't focus. My eyes kept landing on the half-drunk glass of prosecco on the ottoman in front of me. No matter how many times I tried to force my eyes back to the TV, all the predictable thoughts swirled around in my head anyway. *You can't even celebrate your birthday without experiencing this fucking pain. How many birthdays have you missed now? Remember last year when you had to drug yourself the entire day because you were in so much pain you couldn't stand to be conscious? This is probably your fault for drinking that prosecco. When will you learn? You're twenty-eight now and you're still pulling this shit.*

I tried to tell myself to stop. I tried to tell myself that I was allowed to drink a glass of fucking prosecco while celebrating my twenty-eighth birthday if I wanted to—it didn't mean that I deserved to be in pain. I told myself that it wasn't the prosecco, anyway. It was the disease inside my body. I tried to remind myself that I had drunk many glasses of prosecco before in my life and had not ended up in *this* amount of pain. But like with any horrible pain flare, it didn't matter what I told myself in an effort to negate the strain of insults I was throwing at myself. I didn't believe them. I was barely even listening. Before long I could smell the tacos. On any other day it might've made my mouth water in anticipation of a great meal, with the assistance of cannabis. But on this day, I felt like vomiting. The pain was increasing with each breath I took. I didn't know what to do.

I could hear my friends' footsteps coming closer to the living room to see what I was doing. I tried to stop my tears and unravel myself from the ball I had curled myself into. I was embarrassed. I didn't want to have to admit that there was no way I could get off the couch. I tried to sit up, but I failed. I wasn't sure how I could speak at all without letting my sadness out. I felt like such a burden. I didn't want to say anything at all because I knew that as soon as I opened my mouth to speak, a sob would surely come out instead.

My friends came into the living room and asked me if I was doing okay. One look at my face and they could tell that I was not. I started to cry. As I felt the tears come out of my eyes, I also felt a lie escape my mouth, "I am okay. You guys go eat. It's just a bad pain day." My brain was screaming at me to ask them to stay—to beg them to sit with me because I was so scared. But no words came out. I was too ashamed. I was too tired of feeling like a burden. A few minutes later, the pain was unbearable.

That night I had one of the worst pain attacks of my life. To this day, I still cannot think of it without panic rising in my chest. I was in and out of consciousness, screaming on and off, and writhing in pain for five hours before I felt some semblance of relief, and my friends were by my side the entire time. I would have gone to the emergency room if I actually believed they could do something to help me. Usually when I have these types of attacks—the type where I am rendered completely helpless and no longer even feel like a person—I am alone. I used to think I preferred it like this. Sometimes, I still do. But every time I think of that night, and think of the pain I endured, and feel the panic rise in my chest, I remember that I was not alone. I remember that there are people in this world who are willing to sit with me for hours, rub cannabis balm on my back, hold my hair back as I vomit, carry me to the bathroom and help me pull down my pants in order to pee, and love me all the same. And when I remember that, I feel some of that panic vanish. Oftentimes when I think of this type of pain, and the attacks that I so often experience living with these illnesses, it's easy to question whether or not my life is worth living. Having friends who love me in the face of the attacks reminds me that it is.

* * *

Even though I do have friends who have been there for me during difficult times, it can still sometimes feel difficult to maintain friendships with people who do not have a chronic ailment—especially one that involves any sort of Vagina Problems. I imagine it's also difficult to be friends with someone with a chronic illness that comes with a lot of pain. Not because the pain is annoying or a burden or a hindrance in any way, but simply because it's hard to know what to do. And since, in my case, the illness has no cure or way to make the pain stop, people end up feeling helpless. This can lead to frustration, which can be misconstrued as frustration at the sick person when it's actually frustration at feeling as if they cannot do enough. This can strain even the strongest of friendships.

It's not that I need the people in my life to completely understand what I'm going through in order to consider them a friend, but it certainly makes things easier when they do. When I think of the people I consider closest to me, it is often people who have similar ailments to mine. The friendships I have made on the internet or in real life with other people who have Vagina Problems or chronic pain in general are irreplaceable. It's to them that I always go on any bad pain day. I think it's absolutely crucial to have at least one person like this in your life—at least one person who *really* gets it. And that's why the internet is so great. It allows those of us who feel isolated in our pain to connect with others who are going through something similar. But I also have many friends who are not chronically ill, and those friendships can be just as rewarding and important.

Obviously it would make anyone's life easier if the people in their lives understood exactly what they were going through and could therefore know how to help, or what not to say. And although it may often seem like it, I truly, truly do not want people to feel as if they have to walk on eggshells around me. I don't want the people in my life to have to censor themselves around me or feel as if they can't be themselves. But I also don't want to sit at the dinner table and listen as people discuss the mind-blowing sex they had the night before, or the three-week trip to South Africa they just went on, and feel as if I have to swallow the emotions these kinds of conversations bring up inside me over and over and over again. I feel like I can't contribute because if I did, my contribution would be that I am often scared to leave my own apartment because of the possibility that a pain flare might sneak up on me when I am grocery shopping in Whole Foods or looking at pajamas in Target. And if I share that, I end up feeling like a burden. Should I be honest about my life and my experiences? Or should I swallow everything down and pretend I can relate in order to make those around me more comfortable?

Ultimately, I am very aware that other people's lives do not have to stop just because I often feel as if mine has. Other people do not have to avoid discussing the things in life that bring them joy—like the aforementioned mind-blowing penetrative sex, or a trip to South Africa where they were drunk for 75 percent of it—just because I cannot relate to these experiences, or because they make me feel inadequate. It is not other people's jobs to make sure I get through each day feeling a little less raw. I know this! But I also know how it feels to yearn for something—like mind-blowing penetrative sex or a three-week trip to South Africa—so badly that you would do anything in your power to make it happen. It fucking hurts. And if that emotional pain is ignored and shoved deep down inside, like I've attempted to do so many times in the past, it can lead to resentment, which can lead to anger.

Pretending these feelings don't exist is useless to me. *Of course* it can be difficult to hear people discuss their pain-free sex lives, their consumption of alcohol, or their trips around the world when I cannot currently do these things. It feels like a knife to the heart. I know that's not their fault, nor is it their intention. I know that the world is not designed to make my life more comfortable. I know that people do not have to alter their lives in order to make me feel less sad about my own. But knowing all this doesn't make these conversations hurt any less.

I struggle a lot with guilt in my friendships with people

who do not have Vagina Problems, and the guilt stems from anger. I feel myself start to get angry when my friends casually discuss their active sex lives in front of me. I feel like breaking my glass at the brunch table when a friend talks about having to use a heating pad for the first time in a long time during her most recent period while I am forced to use mine every single day of my life. I feel the urge to run down the mountain and away from the hike I am on with my friends when one of them complains about how hard dating has been. I retain so much anger, so much sadness, and then so, so much remorse.

For a long time, I didn't know how to process this. So most of the time . . . I just didn't. I knew, somewhere deep down, that I wasn't *really* mad at my friends. I was mad that I had to live with more pain than the average person, and that I wasn't ever given a goddamn reason why, and that, despite my best efforts, I couldn't seem to do anything to make it better. In fact, as I got older, it only seemed to be getting worse. I would tell myself that it could be even harder to deal with, that I actually lead an extremely privileged life despite everything, but the feelings would still be there. The anger would rear its ugly head, take up space in my thoughts, and feed my feelings of resentment. And then I would berate myself for days. *What the hell is wrong with you, Lara? Are other people not allowed to experience pain now? Dating is hard for everyone; do you really think you're the only one struggling just because you can't have fucking penetrative sex? Periods suck no matter what; other people are allowed to be upset, too.*

But should they vent about having to use a heating pad for the first time around me, a person who has had such bad periods since age fourteen that I routinely ended up in the hospital or passed out? It's a question that most of the time I think I have an answer for: *Yes, of course they should.* Ninety percent of the time I am firm in that. And I want them to! Being able to talk about your life with someone else, without having to censor yourself, is a large part of friendship. But the other 10 percent of the time, I feel conflicted. The other 10 percent of the time can sometimes feel like a personal attack.

I mostly try to ignore the 10 percent of the time when I feel anger and resentment toward my friends, in part because I'm truly ashamed to feel this way and in part because it's challenging to discuss without coming off like an asshole. I rarely discuss these feelings publicly—or at all. Like I said, I avoided talking about it in general for a long time. I didn't even bring it up to my therapist for fear of what she might think. I was scared that if I admitted how I really felt sometimes, and divulged the way my hands start to shake when a friend who does not have a chronic illness says that they understand my pain, the whole world would know what a dick I am. They would then know how undeserving I am, and how my chronic illnesses have not only taken basic activities from me, they've taken my kindness and compassion for others as well.

Maybe I am an asshole. Maybe it is deeply unfair and selfish of me to feel anger about a friend wanting to express pain to me. I can acknowledge that. But if we're being honest here—and I am doing my best to be, brutally so—it still bothers me when my friends without Vagina Problems talk about their pain. It doesn't matter how many times I tell myself I am being an asshole, or how much I try to ignore the hurt and anger I very much feel that 10 percent of the time, trying to push it deep down inside me, it still bothers me.

Pain is pain. I know that. And *everyone* deserves for their pain to be acknowledged, and to be listened to, especially my friends. But sometimes it can feel as if there's pain . . . and then there's Vagina Problems. And living with Vagina Problems isn't just unbearable, it will break you. It will slowly tear you apart from the inside out day after day after day, and just when you think you cannot possibly take it anymore, you might have an okay pain day and go to brunch with your friends, where you are part of a conversation about the great sex they had all weekend. And even when you plead with yourself for it not to, this feels like a personal attack. It feels as if they're taking the butter knife that was served with their avocado toast and slowly stabbing you in the back with it repeatedly. And then, when you realize that you're angry at your friend simply for having great sex, you take the knife and stab your own back.

It's a vicious cycle, like most things with chronic pain are. So . . . what do you do? Do you tell your friend how hard it is to hear about their periods? Do you risk sounding like the asshole you feel yourself becoming somewhere inside just to escape this conversation? Or do you grit your teeth and bear it because you know deep down, without a doubt, that no part of them is trying to hurt you? In fact, on many levels they're probably trying to connect with you. And because you know in the end, you're the one somehow hurting yourself?

Instead of pretending I don't have these feelings—the anger, resentment, jealousy, any of it—I acknowledge it now. And I don't just acknowledge it; I do my best to unpack the root cause. Because honestly, I think we all know that it's not really about my friends, or the way they talk about their sex lives or the heating pad they used during a period one time. It never really has been. It's always been about me and my pain. Although I sometimes feel as if my pain is all I am—all

I talk or think about—I imagine it doesn't appear this way to my friends. Even though I feel as if I've explained how painful drinking alcohol can be for me 96,784 times, that doesn't mean that my friends who are not dealing with a chronic illness register that information in the same way. Vagina Problems are complicated. Even for those of us living with them, there is no easy guidebook on how to deal with these issues and what will affect them the most. So it's unfair and unrealistic to expect that the person who is not living with Vagina Problems will recall that hiking is difficult for me during this day of my cycle because of the way my ovaries feel.

I think a lot of the issues I feel in my friendships with people who are not sick can be boiled down to a relatively simple explanation: As a person with chronic illnesses, I constantly feel like a burden and therefore often am too ashamed to ask for what I truly need out of my friendships. Then, because I do not feel comfortable asking, and they understandably do not remember every detail of the illness that *they themselves do not have*, I begin to assume they just don't care. In the weird way that human brains and emotions work, I've found that it sometimes feels easier to be angry or upset with friends than to humble myself and ask for help. How many times can you ask your friends to stay in with you and not go out drinking? How many times can you ask them to choose a place to eat dinner that has things you can eat without causing you more pain? How many times can you ask for things that make your life more comfortable without feeling like you are always making things about yourself?

The truth is, I don't think my friends would mind if I were to speak up and express what I need to feel more supported or comfortable. Why would they? I certainly wouldn't if the roles were reversed. But when my whole existence feels like a burden, asking for even more help isn't as easy as it may seem. I often don't want to acknowledge my illnesses. I don't want to have to ask for special treatment or beg my friends to come over to my apartment and walk my dog because I am in too much pain to get out of bed. But I do not have any other choice. In order to live a life that is comfortable for me, I require help. All of us do, really. And if I can't ask my friends for help, what is the point of those friendships?

If you asked me right now to imagine scenarios in which I have felt like my friends who do not have Vagina Problems or related conditions left me feeling misunderstood, I could come up with at least twenty examples on the spot, all of which are vivid in my mind. I can picture them with great detail—so much so that it's almost as if I'm still there, sitting at the dinner table, trying not to drop my glass of water due to my shaking hands when the conversation once again turns to sex. It's a tricky thing. It's not that I am not happy for my friends, or that I don't want to hear about their escapades, sexual or not. It's more that in order for me to be able to hear these stories and watch as they move through life more carelessly than I've ever been able to, I have had to figure out how to navigate my anger and sadness at not being able to do the same. I must channel it elsewhere so that it is not channeled toward them. It's rarely ever about my friends, and almost always about me and the limitations I face on a daily basis. I have anger about those limitations. And it can be difficult to be around people who do not have those same limitations. Because no matter how hard they try to understand and sympathize, they'll never *truly* get it. And I think for a long time, I thought that was what I needed in order to form a real friendship with someone.

But what I've realized over the past few years is that someone does not have to know what my pain feels like to be my friend. I don't need people to be inside my body, experiencing the discomfort I feel every day. I don't even need them to meet me halfway. I just need them to be there. I need people to be willing to say, "Hey, I don't know what you're going through, but I'm here. And I'm not going anywhere." And on the flip side, I've realized that I need to be willing to say to people, "Hey, this is what I need. I can't get out of bed today. Can you walk my dog? Can you bring me food? Can you come watch TV with me so that I don't feel so isolated while I'm going through this pain flare?" I have to be willing to ask for help.

What I have learned, above all else, in being friends with people who do not have a chronic illness (or Vagina Problems specifically) is that we cannot expect people to know how to help us. We cannot expect people to know what to say, or what to do, or how to be there for us. We cannot expect people to understand exactly what this is like. It's just not realistic. This does not, however, mean that they do not care or do not want to give you exactly what you need. People are not psychic. They need help knowing how to help. And if we are willing to give people the tools to help us, they will.

The bottom line is this: Your friends who do not have the same pain that you have will never understand what it is like to live with it. It won't matter how many times you explain the pain to them, or how often they see you in the midst of it—they will not get it. But what I have also learned is that we *don't need them to.* We do not need someone to understand exactly what it feels like for your own body to rebel against you in order to be a good friend. It's true that no amount of sympathy or empathy is ever going to replace someone who truly understands what it's like to live with chronic illnesses and pain. Early on after my diagnoses, I acted as a support group leader for people with vaginismus and vulvodynia, and I later started a support group for people with endometriosis as well. The level of understanding in situations like that cannot be replaced. But someone doesn't have to understand it completely in order to be there for you.

And I think I can speak for most people with chronic illnesses when I say that we don't even want or expect people to understand what it's like. How could they? It goes both ways. There will be things in their lives that we could never understand or wrap our minds around either. We don't need complete understanding from our friends. We don't need them to magically know what to say or do. We just need them to be there. We just want to know that people care, and that they aren't going anywhere. We need to know that they're trying to understand, they're willing to listen when we speak about it, and they're not going anywhere when we do.

I know that it feels unfair, the cards we have been dealt. And it feels even more so when we then have to turn around and teach the world, and the people in our lives, how to be around us in a way that doesn't make our mere existence even more painful and uncomfortable than it already is. It's hard, and it's unrelenting, and it's tiresome. But it's also necessary, rewarding, and, most of the time, absolutely worth it. People, our friends, the people in our lives . . . they want to be good. We have to learn how to give them a chance to do so.

I have spent too much of my life being afraid to ask for what I need from my friends. I didn't want to upset them or seem like a burden. And honestly, sometimes, there's been a part of me that would think, "They should know what I need. We've been through this a thousand times before." These days when these thoughts creep in, I remind myself: People are not psychic. People are not perfect. I AM ALSO NOT PERFECT! I am not always there for my friends in the way they need. But that's not what matters. What matters is that they want to be there. They are willing to listen and learn and do what I need. And that is what friendship is truly about—Vagina Problems or not.

9

You Can Still Be a Boss When Your Vagina Hurts

There was a recent study about endometriosis and the effects it has on the workforce of the United States. The Oxford University Press's *Human Reproduction Update* reported that, "Endometriosis imposes a substantial economic burden on society, mainly related to productivity loss." The study attempted to calculate both how much labor and how many hours of work are lost due to people suffering with endometriosis, and what it costs the United States annually. To the surprise of absolutely no one living with this illness, the study concluded that it was a lot. In the United States alone, people with endometriosis lose an average of ten hours of work per week, due to a combination of doctor's appointments and pain. And the actual cost to the nation in dollar amount? The study estimated it was around $119 billion annually. That is a lot of money. This isn't the fault of the people living with this disease, of course, but of the medical system and the lack of serious attention paid to this illness in particular. The findings of this study were meant to shed light on the serious ramifications of an untreated illness like endometriosis, and the effects it has not only on the people suffering with it, but on society as a whole.

Clearly, for all intents and purposes, endometriosis is a public health crisis. And when something this widespread and this detrimental isn't treated with the seriousness it deserves, we all lose. If almost two hundred million people (and counting) in the world, and around 20 percent of the female population of the United States, are unable to get out of bed multiple times a month, and are given few to no treatment options to rectify this, where does that leave us? When the best treatment option available is rarely covered by insurance and costs thousands of dollars out of pocket with weeks of recovery time, where does that leave us? Are we supposed to choose between our job, which pays the medical bills, and living in immense pain without treatment every single day? What happens to people, probably the majority of sufferers, who are not fortunate enough to have understanding bosses or jobs like mine that allow them to take sick days without ramifications? What of those who don't have insurance at all and therefore no access to what treatments are available unless they pay enormous costs out of pocket? Even someone like me, who has health insurance and a well-paying job, cannot outright afford the only surgery that has *any* sort of success rate in treating endometriosis—because it is not covered by insurance and costs *thousands* of dollars. I have to have outside financial help. Many people living with this disease do not have outside financial help available to them. This is not okay.

According to the US Department of Labor, the average number of paid sick days in the US usually corresponds directly with years of service at a company. Therefore, they estimate that the average for workers in private industry is seven sick days per year with one to five years of service. Employees who have five to ten years of service get eight to ten sick days a year. Of course, it's much less than this in many industries, and that assumes you have a supervisor who honors sick leave and doesn't punish employees for using it. And all this doesn't even begin to approach enough sick leave for people living with a chronic illness.

Endometriosis isn't just affecting those of us in pain—it's affecting the world, but it's not treated as if it is. To this day, this condition is still treated like it is just mild period cramps or occasional discomfort in our vaginas. It's as if we should all just be able to take an Advil and go about our day. As if this illness isn't debilitating—both physically and mentally. But it is. And unless the medical industry, and the world as a whole, wakes up and recognizes the seriousness of this condition, it will only get worse. If companies don't care about their employees' lives being ruined, then I assume they can at least care about the bottom line. And the bottom line with endometriosis is this: If it is not taken seriously and given the research and funding it deserves, we all lose.

* * *

The side of my cheek was starting to go numb. I had been lying on the floor of my office's single-person bathroom for what felt like three hours. It had really only been a few minutes, I thought, but keeping track of time was hard at the moment. I was on the ground, curled on one side—the easiest position for me to clutch my abdomen—with my cheek pressed to the cold tile. I could feel a drop of sweat slide off my forehead onto my cheek and I watched it out of the corner of my eye as it eventually slid onto the cold floor. My body felt like it was on fire, but I was also shaking as if I were standing outside during a Midwest winter in only shorts and a tank top. I was doing my best to remember how to breathe. I had a pretty important meeting with my boss that afternoon, but the unexpected burning in my abdomen that had been lingering all day had suddenly flared to a level I could no longer ignore.

I had stumbled into the bathroom, not knowing where else to go and because it was literally right next to my desk, and knowing I could no longer keep the hot tears from spilling out. I closed the bathroom door behind me and locked it. Before I knew it, I could no longer stand, so I ended up on the floor. The same floor that had seen hundreds of my coworkers' shoes and millions of poop particles over the last year. But I didn't care. I would've laid down directly in my coworker's shit if it meant I could lie down and stay still while the burning flared inside me. I was clutching my abdomen in both hands with all my might, hoping that if I squeezed it hard enough, I could distract myself from the burning acid that was swimming inside of it.

I didn't know how I was going to make it to my meeting—or ever get up again, for that matter. My legs felt heavy, like they weighed a thousand pounds each. I began crying harder, and before long, I was hyperventilating and on the cusp of a panic attack. I tried telling myself to stay calm, like I do every time something like this happens, but trying to stay calm when you think you might take your last breath on the dirty floor of your work bathroom is harder than it seems. *Breathe. In. Out. Breathe. You can do this. You've done it so many times. You can do this.* As the meeting time grew closer and my pain showed no signs of disappearing, I became more and more frantic.

It's not that I even cared that much about the meeting in that moment—I honestly didn't. I'm not sure how you're supposed to care about *anything* when your body is revolting against you and causing such agony. I could hardly keep my mind focused on breathing, let alone on a meeting. But I was worried what my boss and coworkers might think long term. Like anyone, I needed a job. I needed income. But most importantly, I needed the health insurance that this job provided in order to be able to afford to see my physical therapist, acupuncturist, and chiropractor—the only things that seemed to keep my pain at bay enough for me to even make it to work most of the time.

The fear began swirling around in my stomach and my chest tightened. The voices inside my head—the ones that always voiced doubt—began their panicking again. My coworkers and boss had seen me at work for half a day before this. Would they understand if I disappeared for the rest of the day and explained later that I was too sick? Would they understand how someone who was able to stand up and walk around only an hour before was now on the bathroom floor, immobile? I told myself they would. (After all, I am one of the ones with a relatively understanding job. We have unlimited sick days. The idea is for people who have coughs, colds, flus, and whatever to stay the hell home and not infect the rest of the office, since we work in an open-floor office layout; I don't think they had people with chronic illnesses in mind when they adopted the policy. Nevertheless, I have greatly benefitted from it.)

I worry about losing my job absolutely every time something like this happens. On this day, I tried to calm my brain down and prevent those worried thoughts from taking up space. But if you've learned anything by now from reading this book, you know how successful I am at that—which is not very. Even if I did manage to find a way off this bathroom floor and get myself in an upright position, how the hell was I going to drive myself home? I couldn't even walk.

Slowly but surely, I began spiraling even further. It happens almost every time I have a bad flare during work hours, despite my years in therapy working on ways to avoid it. It'll start with a simple thought like, "I'm going to have to miss another meeting," and then it grows and grows like dandelions during summer until my brain is forcing me to remember every single meeting, workday, work trip, or other obligation I have had to miss. And once these memories trickle into my brain, I begin to see the faces of my coworkers and superiors. In my mind, they don't believe my pain. In my mind, they all think I am a lazy employee who barely pulls her weight. In my mind, I'm seconds away from being fired.

The sobs were starting to come harder now, and the meeting was due to start in just four minutes, according to my phone. My chest grew even tighter, and suddenly I could no longer breathe. It felt as if my lungs were constricting and I was going to suffocate. My hands were tingling, my body felt like it was floating. I wanted to pass out. I begged for it. If my legs didn't feel like they weighed a thousand pounds each I might have tried to knock myself out by hitting my head on the bathroom sink. I was begging my body to just let me go comatose. I wanted anything . . . *anything* to get rid of the pain.

Years of medical professionals and other people in my life doubting the severity of my pain made my desire to lose consciousness and be free of the pain momentarily even stronger. *Maybe if I just pass out, they will have no choice but to believe my pain. If I'm not conscious, how could I make it to a meeting at all? Being unconscious is probably more believable to them than me suddenly being unable to walk after they saw me at work all morning.* It was now 2 P.M. and the meeting had started. I could imagine the messages from my boss and coworkers already, wondering where I was, why I wasn't there yet.

I was helpless. It's a terrifying feeling. In these moments, I sometimes try to picture future meetings—or life events in general—to give myself a sense of peace. I had made it through countless meetings, life events, and big projects at work before; surely, I would make it through many more again, once the pain passed. But on days like this, the vision is always the same: me in pain. That's it. Nothing else. I cannot see a future or a past. I can only see the pain, and it is all-consuming. Ultimately, I know that I can't live my life this way long-term—not having the capacity to care about the little things. Eventually I have to find a way to care about work meetings, or brunch with friends, or check-ins with my direct reports while in pain in order to lead a semi-functional life. But when the pain gets this bad, there is no caring about anything else. My brain only has the capacity for one thought, and that thought is: "Please, please just let this pain stop."

I don't know how long I lay there on that floor, breathing in poop particles and coating the tiles in my tears, but I do know that I eventually managed to breathe again. And after a while, the four CBD pills I had quickly swallowed when I first felt the tinge of a flare during lunch finally kicked in enough that I was able to lift my head off the ground. Eventually I half crawled and half walked myself back to my desk.

According to the clock on my computer, it was 2:47 P.M. The meeting was technically still happening and would be for another thirteen minutes. I had the thought, for a brief moment, that maybe I should make my way over to the conference room. I could offer my apologies and catch the last of the meeting. But the longer I stood at my desk, hand on my chair because I still didn't have the energy to stand upright, the more and more exhausted my body felt. I might have been feeling better, but I still wasn't feeling good. I packed up my computer. I do this every day, despite rarely using it at home, simply because I *never* know how I am going to feel, and I like having it with me in case I can't make it out of bed. I grabbed my keys, my phone, and my bag, and I quietly stumbled out of the office. I don't know if anyone saw me. I felt like I was look-ing at my life through another person's eyes. I was exhausted, both physically and emotionally. Even if someone had said something to me, I doubt I would have been able to carry on a conversation. I didn't feel like a person. I felt like a body gliding along—and a useless one at that.

As I slowly made my way out of the office and walked the short distance to my car, I felt the familiar sensation of guilt creep into my thoughts. *Was I a bad employee for leaving? Now that I was feeling a teeny bit better, should I stay and try to meet with my boss to explain the situation? Should I finish out the workday?* The thought of going back and sitting at my desk for another minute felt absolutely impossible. I could still barely walk, and it would take all my energy to get myself to my car and home to my heating pad and stash of weed. But I also needed a job, and though I wasn't missing meetings every single day or anything, each time it happened I worried someone would finally realize I was sick and want to eliminate my position immediately.

When I got to my car I collapsed into the driver's seat and mentally prepared myself to make the drive home. I was so tired of playing this game. I was tired of berating myself every time I needed to call it a day and get the hell out of the of-fice. I told myself the same thing I tell myself every time this happens—that if anyone else had experienced the amount of pain that I had just experienced, there was no way they would be sticking around to finish out the day. I told myself that while I loved my job and did think it was important, I wasn't a doctor performing surgery on patients; I could go home and miss a meeting and the world as we knew it would continue. My health came first.

I always tried to tell myself these things, but I only believed it about 20 percent of the time. It was something that my therapist and I had worked on together. I mean, we're still working on it, if I'm being honest. *Lara*, she would say, *it's important for you to be on your own side. When you're already in that amount of pain, berating yourself and entertaining feelings of guilt will only end up making you feel worse and prolonging your pain flare.* She's right, of course, but like literally anything in life, changing that is easier said than done.

Despite the massive amount of guilt I felt at leaving before the workday had finished, I was in my car, and I was going home. I had to. As soon as I got to my car, I immediately felt a heavy weight lift off my shoulders. I felt like I could breathe again. In just a twenty-minute drive, I would be home with my dog. I would be able to take off my pants so that nothing was touching my abdomen. I wouldn't have to pretend any longer that I wasn't in a massive amount of pain. I would be able to cry as loud and for as long as I needed to. I would finally be able to smoke so much weed that I no longer had the ability to feel guilty or even form sentences. And then I would likely fall asleep and eventually wake up in less pain. At least I hoped.

There's a common sentiment in our culture that celebrates "never taking a sick day." Awards were given out in my middle school and high school for students who had perfect attendance. And coworkers and bosses chat openly about their abundance of paid time off and lack of sick days, as if it's something worth bragging about. I often think about the scene from *The Office* in season two, episode eight, "Performance Review." Dwight Schrute is rallying for a raise. As he's speaking to his supervisors, he's going through all the reasons he deserves a pay increase. One of his main reasons is that he has "never missed a day due to illness, even when I had walking pneumonia." Obviously, *The Office* isn't exactly the gatekeeper on how to act in a professional job setting, but the thought process isn't that far-fetched. Taking a sick day is often looked down upon in this country. It is treated like something you should be ashamed of doing instead of something that should be applauded. It is looked at as a weakness instead of as something that should be the norm. People get sick.

But when you have a chronic illness and are always "sick," taking a sick day is an interesting concept. It's hard for me to determine when I should actually take a sick day versus when I should tough it out in case the pain is worse tomorrow or the next day. It's never an easy decision to make—and I think I can speak for most people with chronic illnesses when I say it's certainly not something we enjoy. I am not contagious. My bladder pain from my endometriosis isn't going to spread throughout my office's open floor plan if I do end up going to work when I am feeling particularly bad. But what will the cost be to my mental and physical well-being?

One of my favorite things I've ever read about living with a chronic illness is the "spoon theory," created and written about by Christine Miserandino as a way for her to explain her limitations to her friends who were not chronically ill. If you ever see someone with a chronic illness referring to themselves as a "spoonie," it's because of this theory. One

day, Miserandino was sitting with a friend at a diner when
the friend expressed that she wished she could better understand what Miserandino goes through on a daily basis. As
Miserandino pondered this, she said she thought, "How do I
explain every detail of every day being affected, and give the
emotions a sick person goes through with clarity?"

As she looked around the diner for any help, her focus was
drawn to the silverware. She grabbed every spoon she could
find, an idea suddenly coming to her. After gathering a decent
number of spoons, she pushed them toward her friend and
said, "Here you go. You have lupus." She then explained that
the difference between being sick and being healthy is having
to make choices and think about things in a different way than
the rest of the world must. People who are not chronically ill
start the day with unlimited number of possibilities, or spoons,
in this case. For the most part, they do not need to worry about
the effects of their actions. However, those with a chronic illness do not have that luxury. They must think strategically
about every moment of their day and how it may or may not
affect their symptoms.

For her explanation, Miserandino asked her friend to describe her day. With each moment the friend mentioned,
Miserandino took a spoon, representing mental and physical
energy, away. When the friend began with getting ready for
work as her first task, Miserandino explained that it wasn't
that easy. You don't just hop out of bed. Not when you have a
chronic illness. Showering cost a spoon, too. Getting dressed
was worth another spoon, as someone with a chronic illness
(especially Vagina Problems) can't just throw on any sort of
clothing and be on their way. As the friend continued listing
her day, more spoons were taken away. And thus, the spoon
theory was born. At its core, it is the idea that although all

of us may start out with the same number of spoons in our possession each day, the chronically ill people (or spoonies!) lose them a lot faster. And without spoons, you aren't able to do much of anything.

I think about the spoon theory a lot, but especially when I'm contemplating whether or not I should "push through the pain" and just go to work despite feeling awful. It's not as simple as popping a few ibuprofen and heading into work. It takes a lot of spoons for me to show up at work on any given day. And on a particularly bad pain day, I have even less energy. Honestly, I don't want to have to take multiple sick days a month. I don't want to have to take sick days at all. I don't want to wake up in so much pain that putting on clothes feels impossible, and then have to worry about whether or not I'm going to lose my job because of something I have no control over. And this is coming from someone who has an understanding employer that even offers sick days at all—let alone unlimited ones. There are millions of people in this world who aren't so fortunate!

Living with Vagina Problems is a full-time job in and of itself. It is well over forty hours a week spent dealing with anxiety and depression and the physical pain at the root of it all. It is feeling mentally paralyzed at the thought of our futures, but also sometimes being physically paralyzed from the depth of the pain in our bodies. It is wondering how we will ever move up in our careers if there is no cure and few solutions offered to us for the very real pain we live with every day. More than that, it's sometimes wondering how we will even hold down a job at all. It's wondering how we will balance the cost of living in the United States in general with the cost of living with a chronic illness that the medical community has few solutions to—and the "solutions" we do have are hardly what I could call solutions.

Vagina Problems are all this and so much more, and they are relentless. They do not take a break or take sick days, even when they force us to. They are always there. And no matter how much we try to fight back or push back on the pain that has already taken so much from us . . . there is only so much we can do when everything is stacked against us.

One in ten women has endometriosis. One in ten. It's incredibly common. And those are the people who have been diagnosed. Like most people in a developed country like the United States, a majority of these people have jobs. Because if we didn't, we wouldn't have access to things like health care, medical insurance, or even the resources to live here. Millions of people are forcing themselves out of bed every single day when they can barely walk in order to get themselves to work. They have no other options. None! And unlike me, in my privileged position of having understanding superiors and unlimited sick leave, these people are punished if they try to take time off. If things continue this way, work will not get done. Lives will be ruined without jobs that provide income and medical care. Businesses will struggle to retain talent because some of the most talented people in the world are living with chronic illnesses. This is not a unique problem. This is not something we can ignore. This is a public health crisis.

Now that we're all pretty depressed, it's time to talk about the other side of this, the side where we give ourselves credit. Because even when it feels like we aren't, *we are doing it*. Even on the days when we are stuck in bed, we are still fighting, we are still showing up. We're still emailing people, or making sure our coworkers, students, clients, etc. have what they need.

We work harder as a whole because we know we have to. We put in more effort than the average person.

I know that I have to take more sick days and more time off than the average employee. And I know that people are watching me. So when I am at work, I show up as best I can. I do what needs to be done. And when I feel that familiar ache suddenly appear in my abdomen, or my lower back, or my pelvic region, I focus on the task at hand and finish it as soon as I can so that at the end of it, I can give in to the pain and go home. I do my best to compartmentalize my pain and prioritize what needs to get done at any given time. Do I still have to miss meetings and deadlines? Absolutely. But have I also learned how to be extremely adaptable and find myself able to handle most situations thrown my way? Yep! Do I still manage to get my work done? Always. It's just not always on the timeline I, or others, envisioned.

Having a chronic illness doesn't make us bad employees. It doesn't make us lazy or a waste of company resources. I truly believe that in many ways, it only makes us work harder. So next time you are forced to take a sick day, remember that. Because chances are that the work you put in when you're having decent pain days more than makes up for any work you have to miss when you aren't.

Over the years, I've done my best to empower myself when I have to take sick days and miss work. I no longer apologize to coworkers or bosses. When I first started my career and simultaneously realized that my endometriosis and other Vagina Problems were going to interfere, I offered up incessant apologies, as if my apologies could somehow make the pain go away or provide a scenario where I *was* able to get out of bed and go to work. *I'm so sorry I can't come into work today. I will come in early and leave late the rest of the week to make up for it. Please don't fire me. This isn't my fault.*

But these days, I no longer offer up excuses or apologies. I approach it matter-of-factly and with no room for discussion. *I have to take a sick day today. I won't be checking email often.* Period. End of discussion. For the most part, I no longer feel the need to apologize for something I have no control over. And apologizing never made me feel better, anyway. An apology implies that I did something to make myself stay home from work or miss yet another meeting. But I didn't. I never do. If I had the choice, I would not be spending my day in bed, occasionally sticking a Valium suppository up my butthole to help relax my pelvic floor muscles.

My apologies and incessant excuses only made the sick days I did have to take early on in my career that much more painful and noticeable. When I didn't receive a response from bosses or coworkers, or when their only response was "Gotcha!," I would spend the rest of the day panicking that when I showed up to work the next day, I would be fired. I quickly learned that it was imperative to be on my own side in these situations. I couldn't berate myself the entire day because then I inevitably ended up in more pain when I didn't allow my body to rest and recover like it needed. It was a vicious cycle—and one that I still participate in sometimes if I'm not careful.

The bottom line is this: Why should I be sorry for something I can't control? It's not my fault that I'm sick, and despite being sick, I still show up most of the time. I get my work done. I do my job. At the end of the day, that's all that really matters. People get sick. Maybe I get sick more than the average person, but that's also part of what makes me good at my job. I have the ability to get things done quickly and correctly because I operate knowing that I am given limited time and energy to do so. I know my body well enough by now to know that it's rare that I'll be given two weeks in a row without a bad pain flare. When I am at work, I get shit done because I know it's only a matter of time until I won't have the ability to get anything done.

On top of no longer apologizing when I need to take a sick day, I also do my best these days to quiet the voices of doubt in my head that question whether or not my coworkers and boss believe that my pain is real. What I've come to realize is that it doesn't matter whether they believe it is real. *I know it's real.* The entire community of people with endometriosis and other Vagina Problems also knows it's real, and that's what I cling to.

10

Our New Normal

Who would I be if I wasn't sick? It's a question I ask myself every single time I am in pain. It's also a question I've never gotten an answer to. Will I ever? I'm not sure. It's a dangerous game, but one I can't help playing at least once a week. The truth is, I'm not sure who I would be if I weren't in pain. Because, well, I'm still in pain. And I have been for many years now. The person who wasn't in this type of pain no longer exists. That person doesn't even feel like a real memory anymore. The fourteen-year-old who didn't experience an almost-constant swelling of her stomach or immense lower back pain after sitting in a chair for just two hours feels like a dream I had once.

I try to recall exactly what it was like, but it's fuzzy. The edges of those memories feel blurred. I remember a lot of smiling, a lot of laughing. But was I actually smiling more? Or do I just believe I was now . . . looking back? It's an unreliable memory at best, yet it's something I cling to, and have clung to, for the better part of a decade now.

It's useless, really, to spend my time wishing away the life I do have for the one I wish I had. But when you're in pain all the time and know that some people just . . . aren't, how do you stop yourself from wondering? Especially if you, like me, didn't always have this pain. There was a time in my life when I distinctly remember *not* being in a constant state of pain. But if you were to ask me to describe what that was like, I wouldn't be able to tell you. I no longer remember. I know there was a time, before my symptoms progressed to the point they are now, when I wore thong underwear without getting a pain flare, but I certainly don't remember what it was like. It feels like a different lifetime. And in many ways, maybe it was.

When you think of the life you thought you would have all those years ago as a young girl, and then see the life you have now instead, how do you accept it? And if you even manage to accept it the first few times you think about it, how do you then continue to accept it over and over again for the foreseeable future? I have such anger and hatred inside of me for the pain that attacks my body. It feels like an alien forcing itself into me and slowly wreaking havoc with each passing moment. I fight so hard to get it out. I beg it to leave. But it never does. It may be dormant for a bit, a few days, maybe a week, and I'll start to forget what it was like. I'll do my best to heal. I'll start leaving the house again. I'll go on dates. But then it will return, and I have to find a way to deal with it all over again. And in trying to deal with it, I once again return to that memory of the girl all those years ago who wasn't in pain. And then I return to the idea of the person I could have been . . . if only I weren't in pain.

I'd like to think that I might be living abroad somewhere. I always wanted to. I traveled abroad twice in college, before things got really bad, and although I had pain, both experiences had moments that made me feel more alive than I can recall feeling at any other time. I often imagine myself sitting at a café in Europe, drinking coffee without a goddamn care in the world. What would it be like to walk around on pavement all day and not experience a pain flare later because of it? Hell, what would it be like to even get on a plane to go to Europe without first packing seventeen extra things to accommodate my body's needs? What would I even worry about? Maybe some turbulence? Making sure my bag was under weight?

I've always wanted to be a person who travels. Honestly, I know that I am very fortunate to have even traveled at all. But what used to feel like an exciting adventure now feels like my own personal nightmare. Leaving my comfort zone is hard. Hell, leaving bed is hard most days. I've spent hours, days . . . possibly even months of my life fantasizing about the traveling I would do if I weren't sick. I daydream about buying a motorcycle on a whim in Asia and riding off into the sunset without feeling the heavy weight of my vaginal pain, caused by simply sitting on a motorbike. I want to get tipsy from too many Negronis in Italy without waking up six hours later from the burning in my bladder and kidneys that is so bad, I cannot walk. I just want to feel free. I want to no longer feel the imprisonment of this body and this pain and be able to make my own decisions about what I will spend my day doing or eating.

Outside of my dreams about travel, I also spend a large chunk of time pondering the dating life I feel I didn't get to have. There's never a scenario where I imagine dating would be harder without these illnesses—I feel pretty confident that I'd have a much easier time dating. If the simple act of orgasming didn't come with the chance of causing me so much pain, would I be less guarded? Would it be easier for me to make connections with people? I fantasize about the type of person I would be to date if only I weren't so weighed down with these illnesses. Because, of course, it's not just the physical pain that holds me back in these situations—it's the emotional turmoil of it all as well. It's the little voices in my head telling me that I'm a burden. It's the memory of every person who has ever told my exes how *generous* they are for sticking by my side, or for choosing to date me at all. I see those faces—the concerned eyes, the lowered voice when speaking to my exes about how selfless they are—every time I walk into a bar and sit down for yet another first date.

But most of what I think about when I think of the person I would be if I weren't in pain is how much happier I would be. I always imagine myself as laughing more often. I see myself as more carefree. In my mind, Lara without pain is an energetic, happy person who people long to be around. When pain-free Lara walks into a room, people's eyes light up. She always makes people laugh. And instead of people constantly having to do things for her, she's the one doing things for them. She is not lying on the couch during a get-together with friends. She is not missing friends' birthday celebrations, and she's certainly not missing her own. She's not sitting on her couch crying while watching *90 Day Fiancé*. She is up dancing, drinking, singing, laughing. She is the life of the party. And when the party is over, she doesn't have to stay in bed the next day because of pain. She pops right out of bed, goes on a run, and does it all over again. In my fantasies, life always seems so much easier without daily pain. And I always seem so much happier.

When I was younger, I used to imagine who I would be when I got older. We all do it. I often imagined myself as a marine biologist or a publicist. I had no doubt that I would go to college and play basketball for four years. I thought about all the amazing parties I would attend and the traveling I would do. And when I imagined myself eventually graduating from college with honors, I also saw myself moving far away. I wanted to meet someone; I thought I would fall hopelessly in love. Maybe I would get married. Maybe I would start a family. I wanted to do many, many things. Getting sick was never one of them.

The thing about life, which we all know by now, is that it doesn't go as planned for anyone. It just doesn't. And it especially doesn't go as planned when you get sick. Although it's now been more than a decade since I first realized I was sick and that something was wrong with my body, I still struggle with the idea of having no control of how my life will be—or even how my day will turn out based on what type of pain I am in.

The feeling of being so out of control of your very own life is hard to describe. It feels so fucking unfair. It's maddening. You want to fight back. You try to fight back! But you quickly learn that the energy you use trying to fight back against something you ultimately have no control over is energy you won't be able to replace. It's a cruel joke: The energy you spend putting up a fight only makes you feel more depleted and sicker in the long run.

Most days, acceptance feels impossible. Not only do you have to reconcile with being in pain, you also have to try to acknowledge what this means for you and your life. All those plans you made . . . they have disappeared. They're replaced with doctors' appointments and time spent on your couch hugging your heating pad to your abdomen. And not only do you have to find a way to come to an acceptance of sorts, living with a chronic illness means that you are constantly trying to heal. Whether you're physically trying to heal your body from the last major pain flare or mentally healing your mind from spending hours and hours in massive amounts of pain . . . you're always trying to heal. And healing takes time. But when you have an illness or pain that is chronic, you aren't given time. You are given a few days, maybe a few weeks at most, in between pain flares or attacks to try to reconcile yourself to what happened. But before you're at a place where you feel at peace and ready to face it again, it comes for you. And then you must face it again, even though you feel no readier this time than you were the last time.

So you're doing your best to accept this newfound misery and pain that is *constant* while also doing your best to heal and simultaneously desperately clinging to the idea of the life you could've had. From there, you start to convince yourself that *there must be a way to get that life you so desperately crave.* The one without the pain, without the constant attempt at healing, any of it. There must be a magic cure somewhere. This conviction is, in part, because trying to accept that something is incurable and chronic is simply too hard, and in part because Western medicine and Western society's understanding of chronic and/or incurable conditions doesn't come close to the reality of living with them. The notion that is constantly shoved down our throats is that *there is always a solution.* Back pain? There's a pill for that. Fatigue? Just take this vitamin every day. Trouble digesting? You just need this fancy juicer! There is seemingly an answer for all our ailments. And when there isn't? Well, you convince yourself there is one anyway, because the idea that there's nothing you can do is unfathomable. So you go on a search to find a magic cure, the thing that will give you the relief you so desperately crave.

I've been down this path now more times than I'd like to count. Most people with any sort of chronic illness have. It's exhausting to think about. It starts out with pure desperation. You think you absolutely cannot do it anymore. You simply can't. You hate the way your life is. You despise your pain. You loathe the extra steps you must take every day in order to get out of bed and even make it to work. The thought of continuing with this life for another five years, or even another month, is honestly too much to bear.

So you find something to cling to. *This surgery will finally be the one that fixes me. This laser treatment is going to be the turning point I needed. This combination of supplements and acupuncture is the missing piece. This hormone treatment is going to make me feel brand-fucking-new. Drinking celery juice on an empty stomach every morning for the next year of my life while only eating plant-based foods is going to change my entire body. I will feel like a new person. No, I will* be *a new person.*

There might be a small voice in your head telling you not to get your hopes up—that you've been down this road before. And time and time again, it hasn't worked. It might've offered you relief for a little bit, it might've greatly improved parts of your life. But it is not a cure. It is not going to come in and magically take away all your pain and discomfort. It is not going to erase the trauma you and your body have experienced. But you don't fucking listen to this voice. Because thinking about this new treatment or solution you think you've found is the hope you need to get yourself through another day. And that's fine. You need that. We all need it. You do the treatment. You spend even more money. You spend even more time. You get yourself to a place where you feel semi-okay. You start to wonder if it worked. You start trying to push your limits a bit more each day. You stay out a bit later, drink a little more alcohol, go out dancing. Then you wake up with that familiar ache in your abdomen and everything comes crashing down.

You berate yourself for getting your hopes up, for thinking this time would be any different. You imagine yourself back on that hamster wheel of pain—spinning round and round and round with no way off. It feels even harder this time, though, after yet another failed attempt at finding a cure. Then one day you think maybe that's part of the problem . . . that I'm always searching for a cure. Maybe what I should be searching for instead is some sense of acceptance. A peace. An understanding that although I will never truly give up fighting to rid my body and my mind of this pain, I'm allowed to put down my weapons and just live for a little bit. After all, I am not the reason I am in pain. Nothing I have done has caused this. It's not the Taco Bell that I choose to eat sometimes when I am so sick to my stomach that nothing else sounds good. It's not the two mornings in a row that I missed drinking celery juice. It's not because I don't go to yoga every single day. It's simply because I have a disease. I am not the sole reason for this pain. I cannot bear the entire responsibility for it. And neither can you for yours.

The truth is, I'm tired of fighting. I'm tired of constantly looking for a way off this hamster wheel of pain. As much as I want to be free of this disease—and I want that so, so badly—I can no longer spend my time ceaselessly searching for a cure that simply does not exist yet. I don't want to continue spending my time fantasizing about a life that I do not and may not ever have.

I don't want to continue spending hours reading message boards about different alternative treatment options, and I don't want to continue spending thousands of dollars on specialized doctor visits. I don't want to give up hours of my week sitting in doctors' offices or going to physical therapy. I don't want to berate myself every time I eat gluten or have a piece of chocolate because countless people on the internet have told me that my diet is what is keeping me from finding relief. I don't want to spend every moment of my life at war with my own body.

I do not want to spend every second of the *one life* I have in a constant state of worry about what I am doing wrong or what I could be doing better. It is asinine that not only are those of us living with this pain forced to deal with it daily, but that we are then forced to be the only ones searching for a solution to it. I am tired of searching. I am tired of getting my hopes up again and again only to have the same result again and again. So I am not giving up. I'm just trying to live.

When I was fifteen years old, my best friend in the entire world died in a tragic ATV accident. She spent thirty-four days in a coma before dying, just six days after her sixteenth birthday. When it happened, it felt like the entire world stopped moving. Everything was in slow motion. But what I later realized is that it was not the entire world—it was just *my* entire world. In the years that followed this tragedy, I went through the grieving process. I learned a lot about myself, about life, about anger . . . all of that. I understood what it meant to grieve. I went through it. Sometimes I still go through it. The month of September cannot come and go without me thinking of the days we spent in that hospital waiting room, begging for her to wake up. And every October is overshadowed by the knowledge that soon it will be her birthday, and then six days after that I must remember the day she left the earth entirely.

Grieving for a loss of life is something that, unfortunately, all of us will have to do at one time or another. But it took me a long time to realize that I needed to grieve the loss of another life too—my own. Or rather, the one I never got to have because of my illnesses. It may sound extreme to some, but allowing myself to acknowledge how great the loss of a pain-free life has felt to me for so long was liberating. I needed to go through, and still am, the stages of grief in order to get to a place where I can continue existing with these illnesses every day. And then not just a place where I can exist—but a place where I can *live*. The most commonly referenced stages of grief are the five identified by Elisabeth Kübler-Ross in her 1969 book *On Death and Dying*. They are: denial, anger, bargaining, depression, and acceptance. They won't look the same for everyone. The order might change, the feelings associated with the stages will vary, but we all experience them in one way or another.

For me, the denial lasted a long time. I would say the first two to three years after my diagnosis I spent most of the time believing that one day I would wake up and simply be free of the pain cycle that my body was trapped in. I believed there *had* to be a simple solution out there; I just hadn't found it yet. This denial still creeps in every now and again. I am very aware that I am sick, that there is no definitive cure, and that I may very well spend days in bed due to pain for the rest of my life. But I don't always acknowledge that. Not acknowledging it doesn't make it any less true, but sometimes makes it easier to deal with. And that's perfectly fine. In fact, it's necessary. I have to find a way to forget the attacks. I have to lock them away in my brain somewhere so that I don't spend every minute terrified of when they will happen again. Sometimes I have to forget in order to live.

Anger is a stage I am very, very much still in essentially every time I have a particularly bad day. But these days, instead of trying to shove this anger deep down inside me, I give it space. I acknowledge it. I don't scold myself for experiencing the anger, or pretend it isn't there. I let it pass through me the same way the urge to go to Target and spend two hundred dollars for no reason passes through me. It's there. It's happening. But it doesn't mean I have to act on it. Feelings of anger related to having a chronic illness of any kind are beyond understandable—I think it's a waste of time to pretend otherwise. *Of course* I'm angry. We are all angry. We're entitled to that! We can give it space, temporarily. We can say, "I see you, anger. I understand why you are here. I will give you an hour to do your worst. But then you must leave." It doesn't have to move into our brains permanently. It can come and go, like that urge to go to Target. Shoving the anger down deep inside is like swallowing poison for me. It causes me more physical pain, drains me of the little energy I do have, and ends up coming out anyway.

Next comes the bargaining stage. This is where I find a lot of my self-hatred and tendency to blame myself for these illnesses come in even though, realistically, I know that I did not do anything to cause these illnesses or the severity of my pain.

For years and years after I first was diagnosed and began to recognize my symptoms and pick up on their patterns or lack thereof, I would constantly play the "What if" game. *What if I never ate sugar? Was it because of that sandwich I ate? Is that why I am in pain? Would I still be in pain if I did yoga every single day for the rest of my life? What if I never touched alcohol? What if I went to physical therapy two to three times a week, like clockwork? What if I had avoided this trigger? What if I were less stressed? What if I meditated more often? What if there was a solution out there but I was just being too fucking lazy and couldn't find it?* Once I started this game, I could rarely stop. I tried to remind myself that it's not actually my fault. It's never the sandwich I ate, or the lack of yoga, or the sugar. Sure, those things might make it worse, but at the end of the day, I have a disease. Point blank. Period. *That* is why I am in pain. Playing the "What if" game only succeeded in making me blame myself for something I have no control over.

If I've learned anything on my journey with Vagina Problems thus far, it's that I have to be on my own side. And besides, if I knew why I was sick . . . would it really make anything better? If someone said, "Hey, it's because you were just born this way, sorry," would I be able to sleep better at night? I don't think so. It is natural to desire a reason for the pain, but I am not going to get a good enough reason why I, and millions of other people, have to live in pain. I do my best to avoid searching for one anymore.

The next stage in the grieving process is depression. I've also very much been in this stage, for many years. I still am, quite often, to this day. Like anger, depression must be acknowledged. I let it enter my mind without trying to pretend it isn't there. I do my best not to let it stay there, though, like with anger.

My depression comes in waves and is triggered by different things. A lot of my most depressed episodes are related to my cycle because of my premenstrual dysphoric disorder (PMDD). A week or so prior to my period, I find it even harder than usual to get myself off the couch and out of the house. I have a hard time socializing. My brain convinces me that everyone in my life hates me. I lose my will to live. I wonder why I am even alive at all. Every negative thought I've ever had about living with these illnesses comes out during this time but amplified times one hundred. This is something I have been working on and will continue to work on for years to come.

I think this is such an important stage of the process to acknowledge. When speaking about chronic pain, people often speak of the physical pain. And I get it. It makes sense. But I would argue that the mental pain that so often accompanies it is almost harder to deal with. I've been lucky enough to have a good therapist working with me for the better part of five years now, and yet I still struggle every time I have one of those days where I can't leave bed. People have often suggested things to me like, "So much of physical pain is mental! You have to right your brain first if you ever want to feel better!" I get that. I do believe that in order to feel physically better, I need to feel mentally better and find a way to get through the emotional toll living with Vagina Problems has on me. But that is not the answer. It is not the quick-fix cure it has been presented to me as. And it's also a very naive way of looking at chronic pain. I probably would feel better physically if I felt better mentally. But I feel awful physically *every single day*. It is not like the flu; it does not go away.

It's not just *one bad day*. It's a hundred of them. It's endless. It's day after day of the same pain. If you make it through

Tuesday and get yourself to a good place mentally and then wake up on Wednesday only to have to do it all over again . . . it's fucking hard. And it's different for everyone.

What I've learned about the depression stage is that communication is vital. I still don't need solutions, and I'm not looking for advice. All I want is to know that I have the space to talk about how sad my illnesses make me feel sometimes. Being able to communicate this need to the people closest to me has helped me work through this stage of grieving for the person I always wanted to be. I don't have a solution for the depressed stage of this journey of grief for the people we could've been without pain, but I'm not sure we necessarily need one. The depression associated with living with Vagina Problems will come and go or it will come and feel like it never leaves.

It helps me to visualize my life one day at a time. I try not to focus too much on the big picture of my life because that tends to trigger my depressive state. Instead of asking myself, "How many more fucking days am I going to have to spend in bed due to my vagina throbbing?" I try to focus on the day at hand. Today is a bad day. Tomorrow might be as well. But right now, I'm just focused on getting through today and being as nice to myself as I can be in the process. It's not a long-term solution, but it has helped me during this stage immensely.

The final stage of grief is acceptance. It's what I'm striving for. Some days I feel as if I am there. I wake up and feel that familiar ache in my abdomen and say, *whatever*, and get out of bed anyway. I see my limitations but also the ways in which I am still free. Some days, however, all I can see are my limitations. One of the most important things I've realized is that these stages are not linear. I don't think you get to the stage of acceptance and stay there indefinitely. I think it's something that you have to constantly work toward. It has been for me so far, anyway. I'm not sure I'll ever be at the place where I can say, 100 percent of the time, that I accept the way my life is. But sometimes I can. And that's all I can ask for right now.

I've done my best to allow myself time to grieve for the life I didn't get to have. I will continue to give myself time whenever I feel I need it over the next few years. But eventually, I want to move on. I will grieve for the person I could've been, or the person I still dream of being, while trying to accept the person *I am*. The dreams I had, the plans I wanted for my life all those years ago, are gone. They are no longer attainable. Even if I do find a way someday to free myself of this physical pain, I will still have loads of emotional turmoil and trauma to work through from living in pain for so long. And that's okay! That. Is. Okay. Although I never want to lose that small kernel of hope that someday that fantasy life, or some version of it, might appear, I know that clinging to the idea of something that no longer exists isn't healthy.

And in doing so, I am wasting the precious time I have with the life I *do have*. The one that I am living right now. It's certainly not the life I wanted for myself. No. But it's the one I have. And in order to live, I have to find a way to accept this. I *will* find a way to accept this. I am accepting it. Because although this life may not be what I imagined it to be, it's still my life. It is the one that I was given, for better or worse. And I refuse to spend it wishing it was different. It isn't. It hasn't been. And there's a good chance it never will be, not really.

Acknowledging this doesn't make me a pessimist. In fact, I think it's quite the opposite. I am well aware of the pain in my body. I am also well aware that it currently has no cure. I am aware that I have done my best to try everything available to find some sort of cure. And I am aware that thus far, nothing has succeeded in the way that I needed it to. It's okay to put down my armor, to stop fighting so damn hard, and to just *live* in whatever way I am able. Because the more time I spend trying to fight back against this, the more of my precious life I lose.

The time has now come to get to know the new Lara—the one who has chronic pain and might still have a version of it twenty years from now but is somehow okay with that. I don't expect to be okay with this every day. But to be okay with it at all is what I need. I want to get to know what this Lara is capable of, and I want to dream new dreams of where this Lara's life will take her. Admitting this doesn't mean that I'm giving up—quite the opposite, actually. It means I'm finally allowing myself to be free. I won't stop taking my supplements or attending physical therapy. I might even still get a crystal healing now and again. I will never *truly* stop fighting back against the illnesses that have taken so much from me. But I cannot keep existing in this in-between—this place where I'm convinced that there *is* a cure out there somewhere, but I'm just not working hard enough to get there. I can't live in the past anymore, yearning for a life I can barely even remember and searching for a life I've never actually experienced. I need to exist in the present, where I know I am sick, and where I also know I've done and am doing everything in my power to fix that.

There are different versions of Lara now. There's "Good-Pain-Day" Lara, and there's "Bad-Pain-Day" Lara. There's "I'm

Going to Fight This Shit and Actually Win" Lara, and then there's "I Am Tired of Fighting, I Just Want to Sleep" Lara. I never know which Lara I'm going to get. But no matter which Lara it is, it's never the one I thought it would be, all those years ago. And for the first time in a long time, that's okay.

11

A Letter to the Doctors Who Didn't Believe Me

Dear Doctor,

I've been thinking about you a lot lately. I wish I could say you never cross my mind, but you do. In some ways, you've been a fixture in my mind for the better part of five years now. Every time I see a doctor—whether it be for a common cold or because I'm terrified I may have appendicitis because of the intense pain I feel in my abdomen—I see your face, and I hear your voice. It taunts me. It convinces me that I shouldn't be going to the doctor at all. It tells me that I am being dramatic, that my doctors won't find anything wrong, and that I will have wasted both my time and my money. It mocks me and laughs at me. I've tried so hard to quiet that voice in my head, the one that tells me my pain is never as bad as I think it is, the one that tells me I am probably not even in pain at all—the voice that belongs to you. All of you. Despite my best efforts, years of therapy, meditation, and journaling, I can still hear it.

In the last year of my life, the pain from my endometriosis has worsened again, and I have no choice but to pursue another surgery. When I think about what lies ahead, I am forced to remember what lies behind me. And therefore I am forced to think about you. Although I do my best to remind myself that this is a different situation, and a different doctor, I can't seem to stop my thoughts from fixating on that year, the one where I realized that something was *really wrong* with my body. I'm reminded of the fear I felt about what it could be. I feel the same fear now, seven years later. I lie awake at night and replay the sequence of events over and over in my brain. The unknown was terrifying then, but because of you, it's even more terrifying now.

You see, I know my body better than anyone, as I'm living in it. Therefore, back then, when I started to feel the now all-too-familiar pain in my abdomen every single day, I knew it wasn't normal, despite what doctors had told me thus far. Something wasn't right. I just knew it. And no matter how many times I told myself that the pain wasn't real or wasn't as bad as I thought, I still felt it. And it still kept me from living.

One time, instead of listening to me explain how intense the pain was and how awful I felt 99 percent of the time, you tested me for sexually transmitted diseases, since I had been abroad. Another time you said that I seemed to be struggling with depression and prescribed an antidepressant. You told me it would make me feel better in no time. But you never fully explained this medication to me. Do you know that it took me more than a year to ween myself off it? Do you know that the side effects and withdrawal symptoms from this medication you put me on without explanation were so intense, I ended up in the ER?

Years later, I saw in my records a note suggesting I was "in great emotional distress and inconsolable." Another time you suggested that I was a hypochondriac. When you sent my records to another doctor, you included a letter with them that indicated that I was dramatic, and that I was lying.

Another time, another doctor, but this time I was told I had IBS and that a simple medication would make my symptoms disappear. Before that, another doctor told me it was because I was on the wrong form of birth control. Changing my birth control so many times over the years caused my symptoms to get so severe that at one point I had suicidal thoughts. Another birth control from another doctor gave me migraines so intense that I would vomit, pass out, and not be able to open my eyes. One time, I was told to just put some Miralax in my glass of water each morning with breakfast—as if constipation were my problem and not a very real disease that was slowly taking over my body. And the other time, when I ended up in the emergency room yet again because of pain? You told me to just "take ibuprofen next time."

At twenty-one, I barely left bed. My internship at the

time refused to write me a letter of recommendation because I had missed so many days. They told me they weren't sure how I would make it in the "real world." I wasn't sure either. I wasn't living. I was existing. And no matter how many times I begged and pleaded with you to help me, you did nothing but tell me it was all in my head.

I often wonder if you've thought about me since. I wonder if you even know what you did to me. I wonder if you'll ever even think about those months in 2012 and 2013 again. I know I will. I've tried to forget them so many times. I wish I had known then what I know now. I wish I had known about the millions of people who live with my conditions. I wish I had known that there was an explanation for my pain—that I wasn't being dramatic or imagining it. But I didn't know.

It was five years before I was told what was going on with my body. Five. Years. The average time it takes for people to get diagnosed with endometriosis is seven years. I guess I should be happy I beat those odds. But I only did because I diagnosed myself.

I will never get those years of my life back. The ones I spent curled up in a ball in my single dorm room in college, pleading with a higher power to lessen my pain while simultaneously begging for answers. The ones I spent convincing myself that I belonged in a mental institution because you told me that my pain wasn't real.

It's now been several years since my official diagnosis, and I've tried to forgive you. I've told myself that you didn't know any better. That maybe you really did think you were helping me. That maybe I overreacted, or maybe you just didn't understand the situation. But the truth of the matter is, **I was in pain.** Physical pain and mental pain. I was suffering. And you were my only way out. But you didn't believe me. You. Did. Not. Believe. Me.

I now know that my pain—everything I was feeling—was real. I know that it's not a figment of my imagination or a side effect of stress. I'm not sure I'll every truly be able to forgive you for what you put me through. I'm also not sure you'll ever realize what you did or admit to any wrongdoing. Sometimes I wonder how many others you did this to. How many other people lay alone in their beds at night, staring at the ceiling, wondering what the hell was wrong with them because you didn't do your job?

I want to let this go. I've spent too much of my life feeling anger and resentment toward you. Ultimately, it doesn't matter why you did what you did. It doesn't matter if it's because you really didn't believe me, or because you just didn't know any better, or because your pride got in the way. I don't even care if you thought you were helping me. None of it matters anymore. At this point in my life, I no longer need your validation. I don't need you to tell me that I was right all along. I don't even really want your remorse. I just want you, and all doctors, to do better. I want you to listen to your patients when they tell you they are in pain. I want you to realize how incredibly common things like endometriosis and pelvic floor pain are. And if you are not equipped to treat these things, then I want you to be able to admit that and refer us to someone who is. I want you to be a person who has emotions and empathy and remember why you became a doctor in the first place. Was it to help people? Was it to make a difference in the world?

Above all else, I want you to know that I forgive you. And in a weird way, I am thankful. I thank you for showing me what a true fighter I really am.

12

The Vagina Revolution

Hey, what are you doing right now? Wanna sext me? ☺

I stared at my phone waiting for a response. I surprisingly didn't feel nervous. I didn't feel anxious or uneasy, or like I was doing something wrong. I didn't even fear rejection. I just felt impatience at having to wait to begin sexting an old friend. Finally, after five minutes or so, I received a response.

I'm at a wedding lol. Are you joking?

No, I'm not joking, go in the bathroom or something. Send me a pic. And tell me what you would do to me if you were here right now.

He went in the bathroom. And that afternoon, while lying on my stomach on my bed in my apartment in Los Angeles, at the age of twenty-seven, I sexted someone, I mean *really* sexted someone, for the first time. I didn't second-guess myself. I didn't apologize or feel the urge to throw my phone away at the mention of sex. I initiated it. I reveled in it. I enjoyed it. I got off. And afterward, I felt more powerful than I ever had before.

For me, it has *never* been a question of whether or not I want to be sexually active in some way. I have always desired the ability to experience sexual pleasure and express myself in that way with the people I choose. Hello, I. HAVE. NEEDS. But for a long time, being sexually active was synonymous with unbearable pain in my mind, so it was only natural that I shied extremely far away from it. On top of that, I once had a physical therapist tell me I shouldn't orgasm anymore. There were no ifs, ands, or buts about it. To orgasm meant to contract my pelvic floor muscles. And to contract my pelvic floor muscles meant instantaneous pain. So . . . just don't orgasm anymore, Lara. Ever.

There I was, laying on one of those physical therapy exam beds, wearing nothing but the Calvin Klein knockoff bra I had found at TJ Maxx the day before, when she decided to bestow her unsolicited advice upon me. I already felt awkward enough being mostly naked and spreading my legs for a person I'd met only twice before. Throw in some random objects and fingers trying to enter my vagina, and you can probably imagine how chill I was feeling about the whole situation. And there she was, chatting with me about the weather in between attempting to stick her fingers in my vagina to work out those tender muscles. There's only so much small talk one can have in a situation like this. *Oh, it's been so damn hot recently. Maybe it will rain soon. But probably not, since we live in Los Angeles. Haha, thank god we have air conditioning, right? Oh, is that your finger in my vagina? Don't mind my tears, it just feels as if you're sticking a burning metal rod inside of me. But yes, it's been so hot outside recently. Let's keep talking about the weather.*

After several minutes of this I decided to mostly just stay quiet. Partly because I didn't want to talk about the damn weather anymore and partly because I didn't know what else to say. *Thanks for putting your finger inside me, I hope this means my vagina will someday not be in constant pain anymore!* I don't even remember exactly how it started, but suddenly we were on the subject of sex. Considering that she had barely been able to stick her index finger in my vagina before I started crying, I didn't really have to explain to her that I wasn't having much P-in-V action. But, like most creatures of the earth, once I had discovered that my body could orgasm, I was pretty into making that happen. So I clarified that although orgasming, aka contracting the very muscles that were an almost constant source of pain in my body, often hurt me, I still wanted to do it. I noticed her facial expression going from a slight frown to a full-on look of disapproval, but I didn't know why. She asked me again about orgasming.

Yeah, I mean, it hurts so, so bad immediately afterward sometimes, but what am I gonna do, you know?

Honestly, I think it would be best if you refrain from orgasming indefinitely.

Wait, what?

It's not good for you. In fact, it could potentially make things worse with the state you're in. It's probably best to just avoid it altogether.

It was one of those moments that made me question whether or not God was real. What, I'm just supposed to never experience an orgasm ever again? What kind of damn solution to anything is that? Orgasming should be a human right. I mean, who *doesn't* want to orgasm? I can assure you that as someone who experiences extreme, shooting pain almost every time I orgasm that I STILL WANT TO DO IT. I was too taken aback to say anything worthwhile in response. I guess it never occurred to her that I might actually want to orgasm, and that orgasming was probably in, like, the top four feelings in the world, right after being able to stretch your foot out again after experiencing a charley horse and taking your bra off (if you even bother wearing one). I was just supposed to . . . not do it? What kind of advice was that? And even if I did refrain from orgasming, how was that going to make my pelvic floor muscles hurt any less on a day-to-day basis? Was my vagina going to magically get better as soon as I stopped sinning and using a vibrator? I was pretty sure that ruthless bitch was still gonna hurt. And what about ME? What about the hurt I would endure in a life without a single orgasm ever again?

I left the office that day furious. Hadn't I already given up enough for these goddamn illnesses? I already lived a life of almost constant pain. I couldn't drink caffeine or anything carbonated, and alcohol made my bladder sear with pain. Oh yeah, I also could barely wear tampons, yoga pants made my vagina burn with rage, and penetration definitely wasn't happening either. Being able to experience an orgasm *at all* felt like one of the few things I had left.

When I was first diagnosed with endometriosis through laparoscopic surgery, my body reacted negatively. I lost a lot of sensation in my vulva and was unable to orgasm for months afterward. In fact, I was unable to touch my vagina at all—or have anything else touch it, for that matter—without experiencing such severe burning that I would then be forced to lie down with an ice pack on my vagina for hours until it stopped. It took me *months and months* of pelvic floor physical therapy, dilator use, and touching my own damn vagina repeatedly in order to get my body to a place where it could be touched without instantaneous pain.

And now I wasn't even sure I had that anymore. It had already taken me more than six months to talk myself through even touching my own vagina. Getting to use a vibrator was another month and a half, AT LEAST. I had to learn how to talk myself through the pain while using it and prepare for the shooting pain stemming from my vagina and flowing through my entire body right after. Being able to insert a dilator the size of my pinky finger felt like I had climbed the entirety of Mount Everest. And after I finally accomplished all this, I was just supposed to stop? All that hard work, all those nights spent shoving dilators up my vagina, despite the mind-boggling pain, in order to get my body to a place where it could FEEL THINGS again, were for nothing? That was it? No more orgasms?

I couldn't accept it. I wouldn't. It wasn't just my ability to orgasm being taken away from me—again—but my future. One of the most upsetting parts for me of living with Vagina Problems—outside of the daily pain—was losing the ability to have any semblance of a sex life. I had all but given up on the idea of pain-free penetrative sex. But the fact that I was still able to orgasm various other ways was my saving grace. It was my life vest in a raging sea of Vagina Problems. And it had not been easy. I had worked so hard to get myself to this place. If I could no longer orgasm at all without making my conditions worse, what hope did I have of any sort of sex life down the line? It was like I could see the disappointed faces of every ex I had ever attempted to sleep with flashing through my mind one by one. Was that now my future . . . forever?

When I got home after my appointment, I flung myself on my bed and began to pout. I was angry. Who the hell did this lady think she was? Wasn't she supposed to be helping me? Wasn't she supposed to have my best interest at heart? How could she, though, if she wanted to take this away from me? I grabbed my computer and did the worst thing I could do: I googled. Besides the obvious results of random porn websites due to me thinking "orgasm pain" was a smart thing to google, I mostly found message boards of women with similar pain to mine describing how these conditions had ruined their relationships and marriages. By this point in my life, I had already experienced my fair share of failed attempts at dating and knew all too well what these conditions could do to any relationship. I didn't need a message board to remind me. But trying not to google your symptoms and read message board after message board when you have any sort of ailment is like trying to avoid sugar the day before your period starts: It isn't gonna fucking happen. So read I did. And as I consumed word after word about failed attempts at cures and broken relationships, I started wondering if my physical therapist had been right. Maybe I shouldn't orgasm anymore. If that gave me even the slightest chance at living more pain-free, maybe it was worth trying. Maybe this was yet another thing that my illnesses would take away from me.

Before long, I drifted to sleep. I didn't sleep well—I tossed and turned and cried on and off. It seemed like a juvenile thing, and I was a little embarrassed about how distraught I was. But when you feel like you've given up almost every part of your life to something, it's hard *not* to sweat the small stuff. And let's be honest: Being able to orgasm freely without pain or shame isn't really a small thing. It was more than being able to orgasm. It was being able to experience pleasure and intimacy in a way that I so desperately wanted. It was hope for the ability to someday have a relationship that could involve sex in the way I so often wanted it to. It was yet another choice about my life and my body that I wasn't able to make for myself.

When I woke up the next morning my eyes were red and puffy, and I could feel my muscles tensing throughout my entire body. I could already tell it was going to be a bad pain day—made worse by the fact that I didn't sleep well and had gone to bed emotional as fuck the night before. After refreshing my Instagram feed over and over for almost an hour, I put my phone down and stared at myself in the mirror. What the hell was I doing? If I had learned anything in the past five years of my life, hadn't it been that I, and only I, knew my body best? Why was I relying on a physical therapist with a four-star Yelp rating to tell me what I could and could not do? Yes, she was a medical professional. And yes, she had schooling and training that I, a person who barely passed chemistry and biology, certainly didn't have. But she wasn't living in my body. She wasn't going to have to deal with this long-term. I was. I couldn't take it. I was starting to spiral. I flung myself back on the bed, deciding that I was giving up for the day. I felt like shit, I looked like shit, everything was shit. And the one thing that I would usually do to make myself feel better, if only for a few minutes, I wasn't even sure I could do anymore.

After several minutes of crying silent tears on my bed, feeling sorry for myself, I opened my nightstand drawer. There she was: the tiny vibrator that had changed my life in so many ways. Like I said, there were several years of my life when I legitimately could *not* orgasm. I think it was due to a combination of reasons. My body expected pain and only pain when faced with any sort of intimacy, my pelvic floor muscles were so tightly wound I could barely breathe, and I honestly didn't even know how to orgasm at a certain point because it hadn't been something I was able to experience before. The surgery I had in 2012 to diagnose my endometriosis had left me without some sensitivity in the nerves of my vulva, and getting to a place of pleasure instead of pain was difficult without those nerves helping me out.

After several months of physical therapy and dilator work the year before, though, my body had started changing. I was seeing a different physical therapist at the time, and she had encouraged me to explore. She told me she believed there was a world in which I could orgasm—and without as much pain. I didn't believe her. I wasn't even sure I could orgasm at all. I also didn't want to try! At the mere mention of sex, everything in my body clenched up. I would immediately begin sweating. I felt like I would throw up. It's like walking into the side of your bed frame twenty-seven times in a row and busting the shit out of your knee each time. You obviously don't want to walk on that side of the bed anymore—in fact, you'll avoid it at all costs. And then, one day, someone comes along and tells you that you could still walk on that side of the bed, you just have to be a little more careful about it. Maybe you just paint a red dot on the side of the bed so it's more noticeable, and you approach with more care. It took me a long time to feel comfortable enough to walk on that side of the bed again. I was fucking scared.

But one day, I slowly made my way there.

I was so out of touch with my vagina that we weren't even on speaking terms. I had no idea what it wanted, if it even wanted anything at all. But encouraged by my physical therapist at the time, I slowly began venturing to the side of the bed again. And by side of the bed again, I mean I slowly started to get to know my vagina again. In many ways, we had to work together. We were both so used to pain that we were completely shut off from the idea of any sort of sexual pleasure. And not only that—there was a lot of resentment.

(I don't really love talking about my vagina in third person because it reminds me of this guy from a dating app who once referred to my vagina as "Little Lara." I have tried for months to forget that ever happened, to no avail. But for the purpose of trying to describe how disconnected I was from my body, and particularly my vagina, it feels necessary to refer to it as a separate being. Because that's what it felt like! I did not know my vagina. I didn't acknowledge it, I was angry at it, I resented it, and I blamed it for so much.)

But that physical therapist . . . she changed my life. She said to me, *Sex isn't just penetration, Lara. There are so many ways you can be intimate and still experience pleasure. Have you considered trying a vibrator?* Umm, no, no, I had not. But was I considering trying a vibrator now? Yes. Yes, I was.

I took myself to a place called Priscilla's that same day, after my appointment. I had literally no idea what I was looking for and had never been in a sex shop before. I had only seen one vibrator before in my life, which my stupid high school boyfriend bought me as a joke from Spencer's in our hometown mall for my sixteenth birthday—after he had forgotten to get me another gift. (I'm still kind of mad about that. And also, it might still be hidden in the closet of my childhood bedroom in my parents' house. Maybe I should find it.)

I entered the shop and immediately felt like crying or screaming or both. I was literally *surrounded* by sex. It was everywhere I looked. I felt like the walls were closing in on me. I tried to breathe, but I could feel beads of sweat start to form on my upper lip. As hard as I tried to tell myself that I was not broken, or unlovable, or doomed . . . I was struggling to believe it while standing surrounded by reminders of the ways my body did not function. The voice in my head telling me I had nothing to offer in a relationship grew louder every second I spent in there. But I was determined. If my physical therapist believed I could have an orgasm, by god I was going to find a way. Where there's a will, there's a way, and my will to experience an orgasm greatly outweighed the voice in my head telling me to get out of the store. I wasn't leaving without a vibrator, damn it.

I walked up to the front counter and smiled at the lady working. She returned my smile and asked if she could help me find anything. "I need a vibrator. I've never bought one before. I just need something simple that will . . . get the job done. But not one that . . . goes inside me. Preferably." I swallowed and felt like my mouth was filled with sandpaper. But she just smiled again and told me to follow her. She took me to a corner of the store. Suddenly, right there in front of me, was a wall filled with vibrators of every kind. When I saw the ones that were supposed to go inside of you and were larger than any penis I'd ever seen in my life, I could feel my entire body tense. I think my face might have turned white because she immediately directed me toward a small, discreet pink one that was meant for clitoral stimulation and did not require insertion. It terrified me and excited me at the same time. "I'll take it."

That little vibrator has been with me ever since. At first, I had no idea how to work it. There are settings that to this day I still don't understand. But none of that stuff mattered after the first time I was able to orgasm with this vibrator. That day changed my life. In many ways, the day I was able to give myself an orgasm after years of pain and agony feels more monumental than my college graduation. Of course, other vibrators have come and gone since. These days, I have two entire shelves in my bedroom dedicated to my vibrator collection. But this one was *the one*. It was the one that changed it all for me—the one that gave me the hope I so desperately needed during a time in my life when I had no hope left. There she was, on that day when I once again felt hopeless, staring back at me. It felt like a challenge. And a reminder.

While I lay in bed that day thinking about my journey with my vagina and orgasms and sex in general, and all the things I had given up, and the ways my life had changed . . . I realized something. When you have a chronic illness, you have to pick and choose the things you give up. You can't give up everything, because when you do, you're left with a life that doesn't feel worth living anymore. You must be very thoughtful about what stays and what goes. It's one of the only ways people with chronic pain maintain any sense of control over their lives. I gave up caffeine and carbonation and most processed foods because they always caused more pain, and I didn't particularly care about having them. I gave up wearing thong underwear and tight-fitting jeans because I could wear cotton underwear and invest in comfortable yoga pants. But I was not going to give up orgasming. I had worked too hard and come too far to have this taken away from me now. After all, it wasn't just giving up a feeling of pleasure. It was giving up a symbol of any sort of sex life that I could have with partners in the future. It was like watching the small flame of hope that I had been working so hard to keep burning for the last five years slowly extinguish.

With one last thought, I grabbed my old vibrator, the one that had been with me for so many years, and I got to work. And when the pain came right after the climax, as it so often does, I didn't get upset. I didn't feel like a failure, or like I had done something wrong, or like there was no hope left. I just felt satisfied.

* * *

It's difficult to envision or even describe how I went from "not being able to talk about sex without bawling" to "sexting guys while I shop in Target," but over the course of the last five years . . . I did. I think after a while of encouraging other people to not be ashamed of their Vagina Problems and to know that they could and still would be desirable, I figured I should walk the walk and not just talk the talk. So I started slowly. Being in a relationship for several years while living with Vagina Problems definitely helped. It was a catalyst— much like finding out that many people don't orgasm from penetration alone—along the journey of discovering that sex is my oyster and there is a world of possibilities waiting for me. I mean, the proof was in the pudding! I was in a relationship where we had a lot of sex despite my Vagina Problems. I could no longer say that I was unlovable or undesirable based on my vaginal pain, because I had been loved and desired in spite of it. And we didn't have penetrative sex. Ever. It was the best proof I had. But when that relationship ended, I felt myself begin what I refer to now as my *sexual awakening*.

Being able to own my pain and still give myself permission to have a sex life was a turning point in my life. It was as if the world around me was suddenly more vibrant. The sky was more blue, the trees more green, the flowers more irresistible. Everything seemed to shine a little bit brighter, and the weight I had carried on my shoulders for so long of my pain and the emotional turmoil that came with it was suddenly much lighter.

I didn't realize how much I needed permission to still feel like a sexual person or still desire sex despite my vaginal pain until I figured out a way to give myself permission. I no longer feel as if speaking about my Vagina Problems and the pain that comes with them is anything to be ashamed of. In fact, I am proud that I do it. I am in awe of myself and the progress I have made over the last five years, every single day.

Sometimes I think back to that girl who was lying in her IKEA queen-sized bed, one leg propped up on a pillow and one hand holding the ice pack to her vulva because it was burning so badly. She was twenty-two years old and had just recently been diagnosed with vulvodynia, vaginismus, and endometriosis. She was in pain all the time. She did not know if she would ever be free of it. I think about how she spent days fantasizing about her future. She yearned for love, lust, friendship, experience, life. And she mourned because she didn't believe she would get to have any of it. I think of that feeling that stayed with her for so long—the feeling of existing just beneath the surface. As if life were on the other side, but she couldn't quite figure out how to make it there. Her illnesses and the pain and heartache were weighing her down.

And then I think about how I wish I could show her what I see now. Because for the first time in my life while dealing with these Vagina Problems, I see a woman who has chosen to embrace life and live in whatever way she is able. I see a woman who has experienced love, lust, friendship, all of it, despite the pain and agony. I see a woman owning her sexuality and embracing her pain. I see a woman sharing her struggles honestly and openly and without shame. I see a woman who refuses to be defined by the illnesses that have done their best to define her. But most of all, I see hope. I see a world in which a person lives with great pain and suffering but still has moments of pure bliss. I see a woman who refuses to accept mediocre medical care, and a woman who not only avoids a piece of cake because the sugar in it can make her pain worse but also has a piece of that cake whenever she fucking wants one.

All those years I spent wondering how I would ever have a life with Vagina Problems, I failed to realize I was already living a life in spite of it all. It is not the life I wanted. It is not the life I would have chosen. But it is the one I have. And no matter how many Vagina Problems I may have at any given moment—I will still live.

Acknowledgments

If you had asked me five years ago if I thought that I would someday be writing an entire book about my vagina (and all of its problems), I would have thought it was weird that some random person was asking me about my vagina. Haha, just kidding. No, but seriously, I never thought this would happen. I never thought I would get to the place where not only was I able to come to terms with the illnesses that have dictated so much of my life, but I would also have the opportunity to write about them so that others could learn, or find comfort, or just feel less alone. I am very grateful. So please allow me to take the time to express that gratitude.

First and foremost, I am grateful to you, whoever you may be, for taking the time to pick up this book. Whether you're in a bookstore (and if you are, I hope you bought the book—support bookstores!!), reading on an e-reader, or you found this in a Little Free Library on your street—thank you. Thank you for taking the time to read about my pain. Because, as you hopefully know by now, it's not just my pain. It's the pain of millions of people. Thank you for letting me—us—have a voice.

Thank you to the best agent, JL, for believing and championing this first-time author who just wanted to tell the world about painful sex, and to my editor, Sylvan, for guiding me through this process with such compassion and wisdom. Thank you to my dear friend Farrah for answering every single question I had about writing a book, and to my dear friends Erin, Caroline, and Brooke for embracing every single text I sent them that said "I CANNOT DO THIS" and letting me know that, actually, I could. Thank you to Noel, my first confidant in the chronic pain world and my rock through everything. Also thank you for letting me stay in your house for a month while I wrote this book and ate all your chips and salsa. Thank you to my parents for never giving up on me and believing me when I said I was in pain. And thank you to my dog, Pepper, for being with me every step of the way and for licking my tears when I sat on my couch trying to write about the trauma that had impacted my life so much.

But most of all, thank you to everyone who lives with any sort of chronic pain or invisible illness. I am only able to tell my story because of everyone else who had the courage to tell their story before me.

About the Author

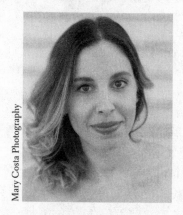

Mary Costa Photography

LARA PARKER is a writer and deputy editorial director at *BuzzFeed* who lives in Los Angeles but grew up in a small town of just nine hundred people in Indiana. She has been a guest on the MTV show *Catfish* and the TLC show *Catching the Catfisher,* and has been interviewed or featured in *Cosmopolitan, Cosmopolitan Australia, Forbes,* and *Glamour,* as well as many other publications. She began writing publicly on her blog, *Outside the Comfort Zone,* in college around the time of her diagnosis with endometriosis and hasn't stopped writing about her vagina since. When she isn't writing or talking about her Vagina Problems, she's watching Bravo and trying to teach her dog how to hug her on command.